CONTENTS

FOREWORD

This useful and practical handbook will help you manage food and chemical allergies through the innovative concepts and methods of clinical ecology.

Clinical ecology began when French Hansel, M.D., became a fellow in pathology at the Mayo Clinic in the late 1920s. A keen and inquiring observer, he noticed many eosinophiles, a rare type of white blood cell, in surgical specimens from the nasal passages and sinuses of those who suffered severe nasal congestion. What did this mean? Hansel, a voracious reader of English and German medical journals, learned from the Department of Otolaryngology that allergic reactions are accompanied by increased numbers of eosinophiles. Could it be that operations were being performed on patients whose runny noses and chronic sinus problems were due to allergies?

Hansel believed he had discovered something new and important. So he transferred to a fellowship in otolaryngology (ear, nose, and throat). He confided to the department head his hunch that chronic runny noses and sinus problems were often due to unsuspected allergies. He was permitted to open a small allergy clinic, and sure enough, he found that most of the patients with chronic stuffy noses (rhinitis) and sinus headaches (sinusitis) were allergic to household dust and molds. With desensitizing shots of the allergic substance, the stuffed-up noses and sinus headaches cleared up without need for surgery. This was a new and original idea—that unsuspected allergy caused much chronic nasal and sinus trouble.

Dr. Hansel opened an office in St. Louis for the practice of otolaryngology and allergy and began to write his book, *Allergy of the Nose and Paranasal Sinuses*, published in 1936. At that time, I had completed a residency in otolaryngology at the Massachusetts Eye and Ear Infirmary and had no inkling that allergies caused most cases of chronic rhinitis and sinusitis.

I joined my father's office of otolaryngology in Chicago in 1932, at the beginning of the Great Depression. Having acquired a summertime hay fever, I purchased Hansel's new book and read it from cover to cover. I was impressed. When I visited his office, his skin testing showed that I was allergic to alternaria, the common mold of Midwestern grain fields. He started me on desensitizing shots that worked. I was more impressed than ever, and returned to spend a week in Dr. Hansel's office to learn his methods, which I then began to apply to patients with chronic runny noses and sinus problems. The results were so good that I became a strong supporter of Hansel's new idea of the importance of unsuspected allergies to dust, molds, and sometimes to common frequently eaten foods.

I learned from Hansel that Arthur Coca, M.D., of New York, was considered the foremost researcher of the new specialty of allergy and that he offered an intensive one-month course in his subject. I was accepted and learned the technique of intradermal testing, which is more accurate than scratch tests to diagnose allergy. I was tested intradermally for foods and reacted to wheat! This result explained my chronic morning fatigue and foggy brain after my usual breakfast of shredded wheat and toast. Omitting as much wheat from my diet as I could (a difficult feat), I experienced renewed vigor and mental clarity.

With my encouragement and with help from Russell Williams, M.D., of Wyoming, Hansel began an annual one-week course in allergy for otolaryngologists at Jackson Hole. I also helped to establish a Hansel Society for otolaryngologists who followed his concepts and methods. This group has grown to be the American Academy of Otolaryngic Allergy with more than 1,500 members.

Hansel was always a keen observer. He noticed as he desensitized his patients, starting with a very tiny dose of the causative substance and gradually increasing the amount by weekly injections to the maximum tolerated dose, that somewhere long before reaching this top dose, the patient's symptoms would dramatically improve. He termed this reaction the optimum treatment dose, getting the best results by simply continuing this exact dose. How do you find this optimum dose? Hansel tried a series of different dilutions. A general allergist, Herbert Rinkel, M.D., from Kansas City, dissatisfied with his treatment of ragweed hay fever, visited Hansel and revised the dilution technique to find the optimum dose. This technique is utilized today by followers of Hansel and Rinkel in establishing the effective treatment dose for all allergies, including foods and chemicals. A remarkable book on food allergy by Rinkel, Randolph, and Zeller had recently been published. Randolph and Rinkel soon joined Hansel's annual Jackson Hole course for otolaryngologists.

Theron Randolph, M.D., an allergist trained at the University of Michigan, observed that certain foods eaten frequently, and common chemicals found in food and water, could cause mysterious chronic disabling illness. Randolph became the most prolific writer on this new innovative concept, which he named clinical ecology.

My research has focused on discovering the high zinc content of the sensory tissues for hearing and balance, and I was invited by Carl Pfeiffer, M.D., of Princeton's Brain Bio Center to lecture on zinc. Pfeiffer had discovered that certain patients with "hopeless" schizophrenia could be cured by taking zinc supplements. This meeting was to celebrate the ninetieth birthday of Roger Williams, Ph.D., the great researcher of vitamins and trace minerals.

Dr. Williams related how he had, at his own expense, sent enough copies of his nutrition handbook to every medical student in the United States. My alma mater, Harvard, refused to distribute the handbook to medical students! These same leading Eastern medical schools—Harvard, Johns Hopkins, and Columbia—continue to oppose the newer and more effective treatments of clinical ecology, including the recognition of the disabling effects of hidden food and chemical allergies. How unfortunate!

In Betty Wedman-St. Louis, you have found a nutritionist and clinical ecologist who can help you diagnose your allergies and start you on the necessary dietary measures to better health and vitality.

George E. Shambaugh, Jr., M.D.

INTRODUCTION

Following a diet after food allergies have been identified is a big problem for many people. A food sensitivity can create an immediate symptom—sneezing, nasal congestion, throat tightness, nausea, skin rash—usually within an hour of eating the food, but such symptoms may not be enough to stop someone from eating it. Headaches, sinus congestion, aching muscles and joints, and low energy levels are symptoms of food sensitivities that can affect a person up to three or four days after consumption of the food. It seems hard to believe that a food could affect the body for so long. This book's aim is to help you understand your body's reactions to problem foods and enjoy delicious meals without those foods.

Adverse reactions to foods are not a new phenomenon. Two thousand years ago, Lucretius, a Greek philosopher, expressed the idea that "one man's meat is another man's poison." Clemens von Pirquet coined the term *allergy* in 1906 using two Greek words to mean "altered reactivity." By the mid-1920s, European allergists and North American allergists were beginning to define food allergies in more scientific terms—for example, reactions between antigens and antibodies in the body.

Today, a growing number of people are beginning to recognize that food may be affecting the quality of their lives and their moods. Clinical ecologists believe that people tend to react to foods they eat frequently. In addition, the grains we eat are usually limited to a few mass-produced hybrid types instead of the wide variety that people once ate. Eating the same foods over and over may lead to allergic symptoms.

A varied rotation diet is usually recommended to help avoid eating the same foods day after day. The menus featured in this book offer a four-day dietary rotation pattern for several common allergy diets.

Food and nutrition are powerful influences on your health and vitality. Your mental alertness and energy level may be directly related to food choices. The best rule of thumb is to know your food sensitivities and eat the most varied diet available. *Living with Food Allergies* is not intended as a substitute for medical advice from your doctor. Its purpose is to help you understand, cope, and live with your food sensitivities.

ACKNOWLEDGMENTS

Many people provide the resources that produce a book like *Living with Food Allergies*. This has been a labor of love for more than five years—researching, writing, recipe testing, and learning how to help others treat, cope, and live with food sensitivities.

Through his courage and tenacity, Dr. Theron Randolph encouraged me to broaden my nutrition horizons and look at food as a major cause of chronic symptoms. His ability to say and do what was right instead of what was politically expedient, inspired me to persevere with this project.

Special thanks goes to Susan Schwartz, formerly of NTC/ Contemporary Publishing Group, for believing in this book. Although the number of diagnosed cases of food allergy/food sensitivities is few compared to disorders like diabetes, more individuals are becoming aware of their adverse reactions to compounds in foods and need the guidance offered in these pages.

How to Use This Book

This book is intended to be a guide to understanding and living with food allergies and sensitivities as well as a meal planner and cookbook.

Chapters 1 and 2 help you understand food intolerance and the different ways our bodies can react to problem foods. Chapter 3 covers ways to cope with a particular form of food sensitivity, celiac-sprue disease. Chapter 4 offers valuable tips on living well with food sensitivities. Chapter 5 shows you how to treat food allergies by providing menus for rotation diets, combination allergies, and elimination diets. Chapter 6 provides diets for avoiding common problem foods. Chapters 7 through 12 provide scores of delicious recipes that give healthful alternatives to ingredients that contain common allergenic foods. The recipes use a variety of grains, from amaranth and spelt to teff and wild rice. These flours have been incorporated into traditional foods like cookies, muffins, and other bakery products for your enjoyment. The finished product may not taste exactly like the wheat-flour product it replaces, but you'll find that your tastes adjust—especially when you realize you are feeling better and have more energy than you had on your previous diet.

There are a number of appendices at the back of the book that provide even more helpful information. Appendix A provides a glossary of food-allergy terms and their definitions. Appendix B provides food family indexes to help you determine which foods are related to the foods you have identified as problems. Appendix C provides a nutritional comparison of flours. Appendix D gives information on using wheat-flour substitutes in your own recipes. Appendix E covers the pros and cons of using vinegar as well as the different types available. Appendix F lists special food suppliers who can send you the harder-to-find ingredients you'll need for some of the recipes in the book.

The book's final sections include a list of references and an index of the recipes by ingredient.

1

UNDERSTANDING FOOD
INTOLERANCE

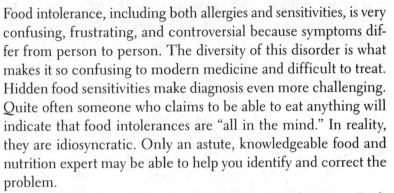

Food intolerance, including both allergies and sensitivities, is very confusing, frustrating, and controversial because symptoms differ from person to person. The diversity of this disorder is what makes it so confusing to modern medicine and difficult to treat. Hidden food sensitivities make diagnosis even more challenging. Quite often someone who claims to be able to eat anything will indicate that food intolerances are "all in the mind." In reality, they are idiosyncratic. Only an astute, knowledgeable food and nutrition expert may be able to help you identify and correct the problem.

Food allergies and food sensitivities are not the same. Each affects the body differently. A food allergy creates an immediate symptom—sneezing, nasal congestion, tightened throat, nausea, skin rash—usually within an hour of eating the food. Food sensitivities are reactions to foods that occur hours or even days after the food is eaten. Headaches, sinus congestion, aching muscles and joints, and low energy level are the common symptoms of food sensitivities. Food sensitivities can create mood changes like irritability and mental fog.

Dr. Jonathan Brostoff runs an allergy clinic at the Middlesex Hospital in London and has a special interest in food intolerances. In his book *The Complete Guide to Food Allergy and Intolerance,* he discusses how food allergy differs from food sensitivity. Dr. Brostoff illustrates the difference with the stories of Jane and Susan.

Jane's Food Allergy

Jane's health problems began as a baby. She had colic and vomited often. By the age of three months she developed eczema. Her mother had hay fever every summer and her father had suffered from asthma as a child. Both complaints are commonly related to allergies.

As Jane grew older she developed mild asthma and hay fever. Her asthma seemed to get worse when there was a cat in the room. Inserting minute amounts of extracts of grass pollen and cat fur under her skin (a skin-prick test), Dr. Brostoff found that she was indeed allergic to both these substances. Her arm swelled up with a red itchy bump where the extract had entered the skin.

Once or twice during her early years, Jane's mouth and tongue swelled up enormously after eating, and she had to be rushed to the hospital. Her mother concluded that peanuts had caused this alarming reaction. Dr. Brostoff again used skin-prick tests and confirmed that Jane had a food allergy and was extremely sensitive to peanuts. Even though Jane avoided peanuts, there were occasional problems. Once when her parents were holding a party, she passed around a bowl of nuts. Later she rubbed her eyelids, and they soon began to swell and itch furiously.

As an adult, Jane had a successful career that involved a great deal of traveling and eating out. Wherever she ate she had to be careful to avoid anything with peanuts.

All was well until Jane (age 32) ordered cheesecake in a restaurant. She had asked if the brown powder on the cheesecake contained any nuts and was assured that it was pure chocolate. Normally this would have been true—but the chef had run out of chocolate that day and had instead used finely grated nuts, including peanuts.

Within seconds of taking her first mouthful, Jane's mouth was itching. Her tongue began to swell and her breathing became labored. She could no longer speak, and as the swelling blocked her windpipe, she began to turn blue. Within minutes she had collapsed to the floor.

Her colleagues were horrified and had no idea what to do. Another diner, a physician, intervened. Grabbing a spoon from the table, he pushed the handle over the edge of her tongue and managed to open up the blocked windpipe. As he did so, Jane gradually turned from blue to pink, but she was still in a state of collapse (known as anaphylactic shock), and her face was swollen.

Susan's Food Sensitivity

Susan, about the same age as Jane, was well as a child. But at 21 she suffered a bad case of diarrhea when traveling abroad.

Although she recovered from this, her bowels never returned to normal. Mild diarrhea stayed with her, and as the years passed, it gradually got worse. Pains began in the lower part of her stomach. When she finally consulted her doctor, she was told she had irritable bowel syndrome, and that she should try to relax more.

For many years Susan also suffered from headaches, but she simply took aspirin to relieve the pain. Just after her twenty-eighth birthday, she experienced a strange ache in the left side of her head only. She took aspirin, but the pain became more intense, and she began to feel sick. Eventually she had to draw the curtains and go to bed because she could not bear the light. More attacks followed.

Susan's doctor told her that these were migraines, and again recommended that she worry less and relax more. Although she followed his suggestions, the headaches continued, and so did her bowel problem.

Over the next few years, Susan gave up alcohol and chocolate as they always seemed to bring on the migraine attacks. But the attacks continued and became more frequent. She also felt excessively tired, especially first thing in the morning, and light-headed and confused, or very edgy and irritable. Then she began to get pains in her knees. By the time she was 34, she could no longer run up the stairs without pain, and she was forced to give up jogging and bicycle riding.

The pains spread to other joints, and she began to feel that there was something seriously wrong; she was ill most of the time.

Susan had previously accepted her doctor's diagnosis that most of her problems were due to her nerves, but now she began to have doubts. She was married and had a good job that she enjoyed. Indeed she felt more settled and happy than she had at any other time in her life.

Her doctor gave her a thorough examination, but could find nothing wrong. He repeated his earlier diagnosis, and suggested that her joint pains were also psychosomatic.

Then Susan read a magazine article about food allergy, which seemed to cause symptoms similar to the ones she had. Her doctor was dismissive, and another year went by in which Susan became steadily worse.

Then a new doctor joined the practice; it turned out that he had a special interest in allergy patients. When Susan went to see him, he explained that a possible cause of symptoms such as hers was food. He also explained why his colleague had dismissed the idea of her having a food allergy—the condition he treated was quite different and he preferred to use the name food intolerance.

He suggested that she try a special diet that omitted all the foods she normally ate.

Susan began the diet on a Monday with high hopes, but by Tuesday she felt very ill indeed. Her tiredness was worse, and she experienced the worst migraine attack she had ever suffered; it lasted through Wednesday.

On Thursday she felt completely washed out, and Friday was little better. In desperation, she called the doctor, but he told her that this sort of reaction often occurred. The severity of her reaction confirmed that foods were the source of the problem, and she should persevere with the diet.

On Saturday Susan awoke early, before her alarm clock went off. As she got out of bed, she noticed that her knees did not give their customary painful twinge. She tried walking downstairs and then running up them again. To her amazement, she found that the pains she had endured for two years had vanished.

As the day went on, she realized she felt altogether different. She was no longer tired, her head felt clearer, and there was no headache or migraine, unlike most weekends. Indeed she felt better than she had for many years. Over the next few days it became obvious that her bowels were also a great deal better.

When she returned to the doctor, Susan was jubilant. Even her irritability, which she had thought was just part of her personality, had vanished.

The doctor explained that she must now reintroduce different foods, one at a time, to see what effect they had. Over the next two months she tried out all the foods she normally ate. Some had no effect, but others made her very ill. Milk, wheat, rye, barley, yeast, oranges, lemons, beef, and tomatoes were the main culprits.

By avoiding all these foods and adding other, more unusual foods into her diet, Susan remained well. Migraines became a thing of the past.

After eight months the doctor suggested that she try out some of the eliminated foods to see what effect they had. She found that she still reacted to milk, chocolate, and alcohol, but was fine with the other foods. The doctor advised her not to eat them more than once every four days.

A year later Susan discovered that she could occasionally drink milk again without ill effects. Then she discovered that she could also drink alcohol in moderation, and sometimes eat a bit of chocolate, as they no longer seemed to trigger migraines. By this stage, she had begun to forget what a migraine felt like.

As Dr. Brostoff's stories illustrate, food sensitivities may be temporary, or markedly reduced on a rotation diet, whereas food allergies are usually more permanent. An allergic person creates immunoglobulin gamma E (IgE) responses to certain foods, resulting in rhinitis (stuffy nose), asthma, hives, and eczema. The allergic reaction can be so severe that anaphylactic shock may occur after even a small dose. Food sensitivity or IgE-mediated responses may develop early in life, have a latent period, and then get progressively worse. An example is an infant who is fed formula or cow's milk and then develops sensitivities to milk and dairy products. Years later, this milk-protein sensitivity can show up as a diagnosis of Crohn's disease, inflammatory bowel disease, or inflammatory joint disease. Repeat sinus infections, sore throats, or listlessness may cause the astute physician to suspect food sensitivities and perform an intestinal permeability test for dysbiosis.

Intestinal Dysbiosis

Since the time of Hippocrates, adverse reactions to food have been reported. A growing number of people are beginning to recognize that food allergies and sensitivities may be affecting their lives. Intestinal dysbiosis, a condition that hampers the body's ability to absorb nutrients and reduces immune function, may be affecting more people than traditional medicine is willing to acknowledge. The mucous membranes in our intestines are confronted daily with antigens, toxins, and nutrients that traditional medicine often overlooks.

Gastroenterologists estimate that the small intestine's absorptive area (the area where nutrients are absorbed and the intestine reacts with foreign substances) is equal to the size of a tennis court in surface area. Bacteria, yeast, and protozoa are constantly trying to induce infection in the digestive tract. This can harm the body's nutritional status. Food antigens are also constantly trying to cross the intestinal barrier for entry into the cells. Determining which foods and microbes contain antigens and create problems for each person takes patience and close observations. Diagnostic testing can help identify the major offending foods by measuring antibodies in the blood that are created in reaction to specific foods. Microbial testing is usually done with a digestive stool analysis.

Intestinal Permeability

One of the major contributors to food allergies is intestinal permeability. The intestinal tract provides an effective barrier against the invasion of bacteria, food antigens, and large protein molecules we consume. When this barrier is injured, antigens are allowed to enter the body in excessive amounts, which can lead to allergic symptoms in some people.

Normally, only small molecules are allowed to pass through the intestinal wall, while large ones (antigens) have a limited ability to pass into the blood.

People with high levels of intestinal permeability, or leaky gut, have been shown to have increased levels of inflammation of the intestinal tract. Antigens pass into the bloodstream through breaks in the intestinal wall. These antigens can cause numerous reactions in the body.

Immediate reactions to an antigen can be runny nose, sneezing, or itchy eyes. Some people may break out in hives or have problems breathing because of swelling in the throat.

Other reactions may take up to four days to be noticed. This may be due to an accumulation of the same antigens day after day as the same foods are eaten over and over again.

If you suspect that food allergies may be contributing to your digestion problems, consider doing an intestinal permeability test. Maldigestion, or leaky gut, may be related to some of the many symptoms identified in digestive disorders and food sensitivities. Jeffrey Bland, Ph.D., has stated that "not measuring intestinal permeability is analogous to not touching first base even though we've hit a home run in diagnosis" of food allergies. According to Dr. Bland, intuitive leaps of faith are made about poor digestion without adequate assessment of intestinal permeability. Without this assessment, the individual with the problem has a right to remain skeptical about the diagnosis and/or cause of digestive symptoms.

An intestinal permeability test is a noninvasive technique using a drink that tastes similar to milk. It contains a large molecular sugar called lactulose that should not be absorbed if the intestine is healthy. A small molecular sugar called mannitol is also in the drink to assess overall absorption in the small intestine. After the person being tested drinks the liquid, his or her urine is collected and analyzed for leaky gut syndrome. This test produces a quantitative analysis that can be repeated in 6- to 12-month periods to monitor how well the person is sticking to the prescribed diet and to assess the person's level of digestive wellness.

IgE Food Allergens

Immunoglobulin gamma E (IgE)–mediated food allergens have a rapid effect on the body through what is called mast cell reactivity. The mast cells release histamine, which can set off reactions in various parts of the body within minutes of the person's eating the food. If the mast cells release chemicals in the ears, nose, and throat, a person may feel an itchy nose or mouth, or even have problems breathing. If the mast cells are in the gastrointestinal tract, the person may experience diarrhea or abdominal pain. The chemicals released by skin mast cells can also cause hives or eczema.

Those foods that cause the greatest number of food allergies or IgE responses are:

    crustacea—such as shrimp, crayfish, lobster, crab
    fish—such as cod, haddock, salmon, trout
    tree nuts—such as walnuts, almonds, Brazil nuts,
        hazelnuts
    legumes—such as peanuts and soybeans
    eggs from all species
    milk—cow's and goat's milk

Known food allergens have been compiled from the limited amount of data available. The actual allergens are the proteins in the food, not the whole food. The identity and etiology of these proteins are just becoming known. The following table shows the proteins that have been identified.

Known Food Allergens

Source	Allergen
Cow's milk	β-lactoglobulin, α-lactalbumin, caseins
Egg white	Ovomucoid (*Gal d* I), ovalbumin (*gal d* II), conalbumin (*Gal d* III)
Egg yolk	Lipoprotein, livetin, apovitellenin I, apovitellenin VI
Peanuts	Peanut I, concanavalin A-reactive glycoprotein
Soybeans	Kunitz trypsin inhibitor, β-conglycinin, glycinin, unidentified protein (20,000 daltons)
Green peas	Albumin protein (1,800 daltons)
Potato	Unidentified proteins (16,000–30,000 daltons)
Peach	Unidentified proteins (30,000 daltons)
Papaya	Papain
Rice	Glutelin fraction, albumin proteins (14,000–16,000 daltons)
Buckwheat	Trypsin inhibitor
Wheat	Albumins and globulins
Codfish	Allergen M (*Gad c* I), a parvalbumin
Shrimp	Antigen I (9,000–20,000 daltons), antigen II (31,000–34,000 daltons), transfer ribonucleic acid

IgG Food Antigens

In the past 10 years, it has become apparent to many clinicians that IgE-mediated immune mechanisms do not explain all food reactions. Allergic problems like asthma, atopic dermatitis, urticaria, allergic rhinitis, vascular headaches, irritable bowel syndrome, Crohn's disease, kidney disease, lower-urinary-tract symptoms, and arthritis and neurological problems such as attention deficit disorder and hyperactivity may be a manifestation of adverse reactions to common foods that do not show IgE responses on immunoassay tests.

Clinicians are now using IgG antibody testing to diagnose food sensitivity, along with serially titrated skin testing with food extracts to identify intolerance of specific foods. IgG testing checks for delayed reactions to food antigens. Clinical ecologists believe that people tend to react to foods they eat frequently. In Japan, rice allergy is more frequent than anywhere else. In Scandinavia, codfish allergy is common. IgG testing can help identify the source of food intolerances by testing about 100 common foods.

Other Factors

Cross-reactivity may be a factor in some cases. During ragweed season, people allergic to ragweed may experience allergic problems from eating bananas or melons, particularly cantaloupe. Others who have birch pollen allergy may react to apple peels.

Diagnosis of food allergies and sensitivities is a process of elimination that must take into account food-borne illness or contamination from bacteria or other microorganisms. An imbalance of microorganisms in the digestive tract needs to be considered as a source of histamine release in the body since it mimics a food-allergy reaction. In addition, foods that naturally contain high levels of histamine such as cheese, wines, tuna, and mackerel may contribute to symptoms in susceptible people.

Lactase Deficiency

Milk is a common food intolerance because of lactase deficiency. Lactase is an enzyme in the digestive tract responsible for digesting milk and other dairy products. If a person does not have enough lactase enzyme to degrade the lactose in milk, the lactose fuels bacteria growth, which causes gas formation, bloating, abdominal pain, and diarrhea.

According to Gary M. Gray, M.D., of Stanford University School of Medicine, the majority of people throughout the world develop low lactase levels between three years of age and puberty. North American Natives, northern Europeans, and Scandinavians may have more tolerances to lactose for a modestly extended period of time. Lactase deficiency is common in people with celiac disease and may even be a precipitator of the disorder.

Cow's Milk and Soy Allergy

A study reported in the July 1993 issue of the journal *Diabetes Care* linked cow's milk protein antibodies in children with Type I diabetes, also known as juvenile diabetes. Finnish researchers at the University of Helsinki believe that Type I diabetes may be initiated in those who are genetically susceptible by the use of cow's milk proteins at an early age. Follow-up work will focus on eliminating cow's milk proteins from the diet of high-risk children. The possible mechanism responsible for this disease development was first presented at workshops by W. A. Walker and K. Isselbacher in 1974.

Cow's milk contains more than 25 proteins, each with potential antigen properties. The most allergenic of the milk proteins identified is β-lactoglobulin, followed by casein, lactalbumin, and bovine serum albumin. Symptoms of cow's milk allergy include: vomiting, chronic diarrhea, abdominal pain, poor absorption of nutrients, eczema, urticaria, and respiratory coughing, wheezing, or rhinitis.

Allergies to milk or soy can develop within days or months of birth, especially if there is a family history of allergies. Changing the infant formula to an elemental diet/formula (such as the brands Nutramigen and Pregestimil) may produce fewer allergic reactions because an elemental diet/formula is basically sugars and amino acids. The amino acids in these formulas have shorter protein chains so the infant's immune system does not react to them as readily.

Goat's milk is not a suitable alternative for cow's milk because the incidence of allergy is just as high. Heating cow's milk does not reduce its allergy reaction because the proteins that are the major cause of the reaction are usually resistant to heat treatment.

Exposing an infant's immature gastrointestinal (GI) tract to the huge quantities of milk normally fed to babies during the first years of life is equivalent to an adult consuming one to two gallons of milk per day. Cow's milk contains three times more protein than breast milk and is biologically designed for rapid growth of the calf in half the time it takes a human digestive tract to mature.

Food Additives

Food colorings and flavorings have been reported to cause adverse reactions in some people. Monosodium glutamate (MSG), sulfites, and tartrazine (FDA Yellow Dye No. 5) may or may not be included on the food label. Food colorings may create ongoing problems because they can accumulate in the body's fatty tissues. Evidence is increasing that they pass the blood–brain barrier. People who consume foods with these additives over extended periods may develop reactions to these compounds.

Monosodium glutamate can cause flushing, sensation of warmth, headache, facial pressure, chest pain, or feelings of detachment in some people. Reactions may occur in people (especially young children) who lack an enzyme needed to metabolize the MSG, resulting in the substance becoming a neuroexciter or neurotoxin.

Sulfites occur naturally in some foods or are added as a preservative to retard the growth of mold. Only recently has sulfite addition to food been considered safe. Sulfites have been implicated as an initiator of asthmatic reactions in some people, while in others sulfites can cause gastric irritation, diarrhea, and cardiovascular and central nervous system reactions. Six sulfiting agents—sodium dioxide, sodium and potassium metabisulfite, sodium and potassium bisulfite, and sodium sulfite—are widely used in foods.

Ben F. Feingold, M.D., identified any compound—natural or synthetic—as having the capacity to produce adverse reactions if an individual has the appropriate genetic profile. Since food is a mixture of chemicals, and many processed foods contain artificial color and flavorings, these compounds can affect neurological behavior. Since artificial coloring and flavoring in foods have only cosmetic value, these products serve no purpose in the diet. You may be best off avoiding them until testing can determine which, if any, you need to avoid.

Medical research has verified that a sensitivity to tartrazine compounds (found in FDA Yellow Dye No. 5) in food colorings can grow from 30 to 60 days after ingestion by adults. Since tartrazine is ubiquitous in the processed food supply—some 37,000 foods contain it, according to a report done by the National Academy of Sciences in 1994—a simple, no-additive diet is needed for those with a sensitivity to tartrazine compounds in foods.

Fat Substitutes—The New Food Additives

In the interest of lowering fat content in the daily diet, fat substitutes are being developed and used in processed foods. Many of these products have not undergone testing as food additives because they are developed from foods that are eaten in the daily diet. Insufficient research has been done on fat substitutes like oatrim, olestra, and Simplese (dextrin) to determine the health problems they may pose. Food allergy and food-sensitivity problems may increase as these products permeate the food supply and consumers are unaware that oatrim is made from oats and dextrin from wheat, tapioca, or corn. In addition, protein components of egg white and milk may be used in these products without any indication on the label.

2

FOOD ALLERGY TESTING

BY GEORGE E. SHAMBAUGH, JR., M.D.

There are two distinct types of food allergy. The first is easily diagnosed by both the allergic person and the physician and results from eating an allergenic food that is consumed only occasionally. Symptoms of a reaction to this food occur soon after eating it so the person usually recognizes the connection between the food and the reaction, and learns to avoid the food. No diagnostic tests are needed other than this one experience. In fact, such a food should not be tested because anaphylactic shock, which can be fatal, may occur from a skin test or feeding test.

The second type of food allergy is quite different. It is appropriately called a hidden food allergy. Neither the allergic person nor the physician is likely to suspect that chronic symptoms are caused by a food the person consumes daily or several times a week. These are some of the symptoms caused by a hidden food allergy:

- headaches
- a feeling of brain fog
- impaired memory
- mental confusion
- chronic fatigue despite adequate sleep
- chronic stuffy nose
- persistent head colds that last more than the usual week to 10 days
- indigestion
- heartburn with bloating and gas

- diarrhea or constipation
- muscle and joint pain and tenderness
- fibromyalgia
- recurrent hives of unexplained origin

These hidden food allergies were first recognized by researchers Dr. Albert Rowe of California, Dr. Wayne Duke of Oklahoma City, and Dr. Roger Vaughan of Richmond, Virginia. Dr. Herbert Rinkel, an allergist from Kansas City, with Dr. Theron Randolph and Dr. Michael Zeller of Chicago, authored a classic text entitled *Food Allergy* that described in detail this common but generally unrecognized cause of chronic illness. Dr. Rinkel made two important food allergy discoveries: a reliable test for hidden food allergies and the rotary diversified diet (rotation diet) needed by these patients to prevent allergies to foods eaten frequently.

Dr. Rinkel's personal experience led him to find a test for hidden food allergy. While a student at Northwestern Medical School, Rinkel developed a persistent, annoying stuffy, drippy nose. He suspected he might be allergic to eggs. His father, a farmer, sent him a gross of eggs each week to help feed his wife and two children. To test this idea, Rinkel broke three eggs into a blender and drank the mixture. Nothing happened. Still suspecting eggs, however, he avoided them for some days. Then he attended a birthday party where he ate a piece of angel food cake and promptly fell to the floor, briefly unconscious. When he recovered, he wondered whether the avoidance of eggs for four or more days had caused the violent reaction to the egg whites in the cake. He tested himself again, and again experienced a violent reaction. Rinkel proposed that completely avoiding a specific suspected food for four to seven days, and then experiencing a definite reaction after eating it, could identify it as a hidden food allergy.

Dr. Rinkel's test has remained the gold standard feeding test for hidden food allergies. It can be done at home by anyone who suspects an allergy to a frequently eaten food. However—and this is important—such a test can result in a violent reaction such as the one Dr. Rinkel experienced, or an epileptic attack or even a heart attack, so self-testing can be risky.

An alternative test for hidden food allergies was discovered by Dr. Carlton Lee, whose wife suffered severe, life-threatening asthma. In addition to dust, molds, and pollens, Dr. Lee suspected one or more common foods; he began to test her with tiny amounts of a food extract injected intradermally at various dilutions. He observed that when a particular dilution of a certain food caused his wife's asthma to increase, a second intradermal injection of a weaker dose could immediately relieve the increased breathing difficulty. Lee, a careful observer, concluded that by intradermal testing of a suspected food, exacerbated symptoms could be turned off by a more diluted injection.

The wife of Dr. Joseph Miller, an allergist in Mobile, Alabama, also had asthma. Her asthma was severe and poorly controlled. After he heard Dr. Lee lecture about his observations, Miller tried the method with his wife.

Drs. Lee and Miller prefer subcutaneous injections of the neutralizing dose once or twice a week for treating food and environmental allergies. Other clinics use sublingual drops of the allergenic foods, prescribed daily, to achieve similar results based on the protocols of Dr. David Morris of LaCrosse, Wisconsin. These treatments are usually combined with Rinkel's rotary diversified diet for best results.

There are also other tests available for food and inhalant allergies. The RAST (Radioallergosorbent) test measures the presence of food-specific IgE in a blood sample. The ELISA (enzyme linked immunosorbent assay) method of testing identifies IgE and IgE antigens, which can be useful in detecting food sensitivities. There is some concern among professionals about the value of these tests in making a diagnosis. So until a better testing protocol can be identified, a combination of approaches— detailed food and nutrition history, a symptom checklist, and whatever analytical testing is appropriate for the individual—seems to be the best way to diagnose and treat hidden food allergens.

Finding out how many substances you are allergic to is also of prime importance in treatment. If a person is allergic to dust and molds or pollens, and to one or more common foods, and to chemicals, the best clinical results are achieved by treating all three allergies: inhalants, foods, and chemicals. It is unusual for severe allergic symptoms to be caused by only one of these allergens. Another factor to consider in assessing allergic symptoms is your level of stress, either physical or mental, or both. Lifestyle changes may be needed to see full benefit from food allergy treatment programs.

Nutritional deficiencies and hormonal imbalances also contribute to the acquisition of allergies. Thyroid hormone deficiency aggravates allergic symptoms. Estrogen and/or progesterone imbalances and sensitivities may need to be evaluated to diminish allergic symptoms.

For optimum health, vitamins and mineral supplements greater than the RDA may need to be considered. Vitamins C, E, and B_6 have been shown to help reduce allergic symptoms. Today's American diet becomes more deficient each year as more of our food is factory-prepared for convenience and increased shelf life.

3

COPING WITH
CELIAC-SPRUE DISEASE

Celiac-sprue disease (CS), also called gluten-sensitive enteropathy or nontropical sprue, affects about 1 in every 2,000 people in the United States. Diagnoses of celiac disease are more common in countries such as Ireland, Scotland, and England than the United States because they tend to have heightened awareness of the condition. It has only been since the early 1950s that U.S. medical doctors recognized that celiac disease requires a lifelong commitment to a gluten-free diet. When my mother was told I had CS, the pediatrician told her I'd outgrow it by age seven. Consequently, she never told me I had CS until 20 years later after I had experienced numerous medical problems related to the condition.

Celiac disease is associated with eating the gluten proteins found in wheat, rye, barley, triticale, and oats. In people with the condition, eating these grains prevents the intestine from absorbing enough nutrients, and can lead to bacteria and fungal overgrowth in the gut. Research has shown that as little as ½ teaspoon of wheat flour can affect intestinal absorption, leading to B-vitamin deficiency, especially folic acid. The poor absorption, called malabsorption, leads to abdominal distension, muscle wasting, and fatigue. In children it is often diagnosed as failure to thrive.

Historical Perspective

A Roman physician wrote about celiac disease as early as A.D. 250. In 1888, Samuel Gee, M.D., wrote *On the Coeliac Affliction*, but it wasn't until the 1950s that certain cereal grains were identified as harmful to those with celiac disease. It was noted that previously diagnosed celiac patients in Holland improved during the war years when grain products were in short supply.

Then in the 1960s physicians assessing disorders of the skin discovered that an itchy rash called dermatitis herpetiformis may be caused from villi atrophy in the small intestines. A gluten-free diet was recommended for this condition.

By the late 1970s immunological abnormalities were considered in the diagnosis of celiac disease. Current medical research is focusing on the genetic and immunological factors of gluten toxicity. Biochemists are working on identifying the amino acid fractions of gluten that cause the villous atrophy seen in celiac and dermatitis herpetiformis.

In the 1980s one of the controversies in CS focused on the use of oats in the diet. Some individuals with CS can tolerate oatmeal without recurring symptoms; but the purity of oat products has also been questioned. Processing equipment used for wheat products may be used for oatmeal, creating a cross-contamination. The use of oats in a gluten-free diet continues to remain controversial.

Symptoms

Symptoms of celiac-sprue disease can appear at any age. In adults it is likely that symptoms have been too mild to be noticed for years before a trauma or stressful life event triggers the diagnosis. There is clear evidence that genetics is a significant component in the disease. Another factor in the onset of disease symptoms is a trigger. That trigger may be environmental (eating a large amount of wheat foods), situational (emotional stress), physical (pregnancy or surgery), or pathological (viral infection).

Celiac or gluten enteropathy symptoms can appear at any time. Recent evidence indicates that it is not uncommon for symptoms to disappear during late childhood and reappear in adulthood. During this latent period, considerable damage may be done to the small intestine, causing the body to be deprived of nutrients needed during growth and fertility periods. Celiacs who do not follow a gluten-free diet stand a greater chance of getting certain kinds of cancer, like intestinal lymphoma, and having reduced fertility.

Like food allergies, celiac disease is treated by avoiding specific foods. Some people have only marginal success at implementing a totally gluten-free diet because grains, especially wheat, are used in a wide variety of food products.

If untreated, or if celiacs continue to eat gluten, they can develop lactose intolerance. Lactose is the sugar/carbohydrate found in dairy products. Lactose sugar needs to be broken down by the lactase enzyme, which is produced by the villi in the small intestine. Since gluten damages the villi, untreated celiacs can have problems digesting milk and milk products.

Celiacs can also have other food sensitivities. Even though they follow a gluten-free diet, they may be sensitive to proteins in eggs or soy, or MSG, or other common allergens. While these allergens do not destroy the villi in the gut, they can cause leaky gut, with symptoms just like those those other people with food allergies experience.

Adult celiac disease is a great mimic of other diseases. Add to that the outdated information frequently taught to medical students and you can see why diagnosis may be a problem. Here are some common symptoms of celiac-sprue disease.

Gastrointestinal Complaints	Nongastrointestinal Complaints
Diarrhea	Dermatitis herpetiformis
Constipation	Fatigue
Lactose intolerance	Anemia
Abdominal pain	Bone pain/fractures
Nausea/bloating	Depression
Weight loss	Neurological complications
Pseudo–bowel obstruction	Poor diabetic control
Lymphoma	Infertility

Gastrointestinal Complaints	Nongastrointestinal Complaints
Pancreatitis	Arthralgias
	Dental enamel defects

Malabsorption of nutrients from a damaged digestive tract usually begins with feelings of fatigue, weakness, lassitude, weight loss, sore tongue, muscle cramps, scaly skin, joint pain, and a protruding abdomen. Supplements of vitamins A, D, E, and K are usually recommended to overcome dry skin and aid villi growth in the intestine. Diarrhea frequently results in calcium and magnesium losses that can lead to more muscle cramping and joint pains, so supplements of those minerals are frequently recommended by nutritionists.

Another nutritional factor in celiac-sprue disease is impaired protein metabolism. Anemia can result from the loss of proteins in the gut. Muscle wasting and weakness can be reversed with adequate protein in the diet.

Diagnosis

Although a small intestinal biopsy remains the gold standard for diagnosis of celiac disease, several less invasive screening tests are now available. Blood antibody tests can help detect CS. Other tests like IgA assays and ELISA (enzyme-linked immunosorbent assays) can be useful in identifying this disorder.

A small intestinal biopsy is done by passing a small flexible tube down the throat, through the stomach, and into the small intestine. At the end of this tube is a metal capsule housing a small cylindrical knife and one or two holes. Suction is applied through the tube and minute pieces of the small intestine are cut off by the knife. The tube is removed and the tissue samples are examined under a microscope for diagnosis.

Treatment of Celiac Disease

A diet that excludes wheat, oats, rye, and barley is the cornerstone of treatment for celiac disease. Small amounts of gluten in the diet may not cause a noticeable reaction or noticeably higher levels of the antigliadin antibody but they can still activate immune responses that produce food-sensitivity symptoms.

Maize (corn) and rice are considered nontoxic and used as wheat substitutes in the diet even though they are members of biological subfamilies that include grains containing gluten.

Debate over how strict a gluten-free diet should be followed causes confusion for many and results in some people being less vigilant than is necessary. An eight-year-old boy whose only reported exposure to gluten was a Holy Communion wafer once a week had poor growth and partial atrophy of the villi in his intestine from that small amount! The debate continues on how much is too much gluten in a gluten-free diet.

Recent development of ELISA home-test kits have detected that some commercial foods sold as gluten-free still contain small amounts of gliadin, the protein found in gluten. Up to 1 milligram of gliadin per 100 grams of dry product has been shown to be present in foods that are labeled gluten-free. No government labeling program (or enforcement of gluten-free label accuracy) exists in the United States, making it hard for people with celiac disease to purchase ready-to-use products.

If certain people with CS do not adhere to a strict gluten-free diet they may suffer from significantly decreased absorption of nutrients in the small intestine. This means that their bodies will not be able to benefit from even the healthiest diet. Diets containing as little as 2–5 grams gluten per day have been reported to cause gastrointestinal changes (100 grams of wheat flour = 7 grams gluten; 1 slice white bread = 1 gram gluten). The wheat kernel is composed of 40 different components and 4 gliadins. Research has not yet fully identified which components individually or in combination contribute to the food allergy problems of celiac disease. So misinformation often abounds in this lifelong food allergy.

Long-term significance of minor changes in the intestines of people with celiac disease are uncertain. Celiacs who continue to consume foods that contain gluten have been reported to have an increased rate of intestinal malignancies, possibly due to intestinal permeability or free-radical damage from the gluten in common grains. They may suffer from diarrhea, malodorous stools, abdominal distention, anemia, and impaired vitamin K absorption throughout their life.

Basics of a Gluten-Free Diet

Stocking the kitchen with some basic foods can provide variety to the gluten-free diet. An all-purpose rice- or potato-based gluten-free baking mix can be used for pancakes, muffins, cookies, and cakes. Cornstarch, tapioca, or sweet rice flour makes a good thickener for gravies and stews. Cooking oils and butter or margarine are used only sparingly since poor absorption of fat is a common problem. Xanthan gum, baking soda, and baking powder are used for leavening quick breads made with rice or potato or bean flours. You will find many gluten-free recipes in *Living with Food Allergies* to make a gluten-free diet delicious for the whole family to enjoy.

Learning the foods to avoid on a celiac diet is a lot like learning to drive a car. There are many foods that can be hazardous to your health just like road hazards can impair your driving. You need to stay alert, but you'll soon get used to it. Here are some of the foods that contain gluten; pay special attention to these on food labels and menus and learn to avoid them.

bagels
barley
beer
biscuits
bran
bread
bulgur
couscous
croutons
durum
flour

graham flour
graham crackers
kamut
macaroni
malt
malt flavoring
malted milk
malt vinegar
matzo meal
muesli
oat bran
pasta
rye
semolina
spelt
triticale
wheat
wheat germ
wheat starch
whole wheat

Eating in Restaurants

When ordering food in restaurants, request that bread items such as toast, rolls, or croutons be left off. That way you'll avoid crumbs sticking to your safe food. Tacos and Chinese foods are not necessarily safe because cereal fillers may be added to the meat fillings. Soy sauce is a big offender in Chinese and Japanese restaurants because many soy sauces are made from wheat as well as soybeans.

Coping with the CS Diet

If you have CS, you'll need to research every food you put into your body. Don't be complacent about checking with food manufacturers, because they change their ingredients frequently. One year chewing gum may be dusted with cornstarch and another year with wheat starch. If you don't feel well, or find symptoms recurring, recheck food labels.

Also be aware that over-the-counter and prescription medicines may contain gluten or gliaden. Ask your pharmacist to check on this for you.

4

HINTS ON LIVING WITH
FOOD SENSITIVITIES

Many people with food allergies are overwhelmed with the changes in their daily eating habits that may be necessary for them to feel better. Whether you are a person with an intolerance to milk, the parent of a newly diagnosed celiac child, or an adult cancer patient whose radiation therapy may have resulted in food sensitivities, it's important to establish the mind-set of learning everything you can about the problem. Then you will be more prepared to set realistic goals on how to modify personal and family lifestyles.

Some families will find it easiest to have everyone eat the same diet as the person with the sensitivities. That way separate dishes are not needed. Nonallergic family members can eat other foods when they are outside the home.

Temptations

After diagnosing the food sensitivities, the benefits of avoiding the reactive foods are usually noted within six to eight days. It may take as long as six months to see full recovery of energy and stamina. Then temptation begins.

The first temptation for someone with food allergies is to start taking liberties with the diet. The person may get away with a little bit of an allergen and think that he or she is "cured" or able to eat the food again. Eating a little bit of the allergy-producing food soon leads to cravings for more. And the allergy cycle begins again.

A second temptation comes when traveling or visiting family or friends. In an effort to not be different or cause more work for someone, the person with food sensitivities relaxes her guard and eats what is served. When an inappropriate food is eaten, there is nothing to do except wait for it to make its way out of the body. The ill effects of eating the food—nausea, migraine, stomach distention, irritability, etc.—usually subside in 24–48 hours. This is a reminder that careful monitoring of the diet is important.

When invited to someone's house for a meal, it is wise to advise them that you have food intolerances or plan to bring your own food, and let others taste how good your diet can be. A major goal of the *Living with Food Allergies* menus and recipes is to illustrate that no one needs to feel deprived following a food allergy diet. You just need to be a smart food consumer and label reader!

Rules of the Road

1. Read all labels and ask questions about how food is prepared in restaurants.
2. If you are sensitive to a food, eating it raw will cause more problems than cooked. Fresh picked foods are more potent in allergens than produce that is several days old. The root or tuber foods (potatoes, beets, carrots) are more potent than the greens (lettuce, spinach) that are grown above ground.
3. Do not eat a combination of reactive foods when introducing them back into your diet. The combined effect can produce a powerful allergic reaction greater than from eating just one food.
4. Prepare simple meals of four to five foods—like the menus provided in *Living with Food Allergies*—to provide good variety and minimize food additives and chemicals.

5. Consume leftovers in one to two days or freeze immediately after preparation. Foods left in the refrigerator for four to five days may contain mold.

Surviving an Allergy Attack

Not every stomachache after eating constitutes a food allergy reaction but you need to take special care to avoid a potential medical crisis. Approximately 3 to 5 percent of American adults and 5 to 6 percent American children suffer from food allergies. That is over 7 million people who may ingest a food allergen that could possibly cause a reaction as severe as anaphylaxis. The general body shock of anaphylaxis may include hives; vomiting; diarrhea; breathing difficulty; swelling of the mouth, tongue, and throat; and a rapid drop in blood pressure. Without quick medical attention, this person could die.

Fortunately, most food allergy reactions are not that severe. While migraines and queasy stomachs are bad enough, they are seldom life threatening. Symptoms pass in 24–48 hours, and the severity of the pain may be enough to prevent consumption of the allergen again.

Help for a Queasy Stomach

It is frustrating and upsetting to watch someone suffering with nausea trying to eat. All the encouragement in the world is not going to ease the discomfort. A certain amount of weight loss is usually expected until the gastrointestinal tract can be restored to better health.

Eating soothing foods is the best way to try to restore some calorie intake. Spicy foods should be avoided since they are frequently associated with allergies and intolerances. Of course, plenty of clear fluids are necessary to maintain hydration.

It is important to eat something even when nausea is severe and prolonged. An empty stomach serves as a holding tank for digestive acids, which can make the nausea worse. Eating small amounts of soothing meals can start the digestive process and help reduce the nausea.

Here are a few tips to remember when trying to overcome the queasy stomach caused from eating foods with allergens.

- Avoid spicy and high-fat foods.
- Do not eat raw foods (vegetables and fruits).
- Avoid milk products.
- Select tuber vegetables (sweet potatoes, potatoes) or rice as the carbohydrate, and chicken, turkey, or fish as the protein food.

Managing a Rotation Diet

Following a four-day rotation diet can be stressful during the first couple weeks. One of the easiest ways to adapt to this new eating style is to take the menu that fits the food allergen regime and use an index card system to keep track of the regime.

- Label each meal with the day and meal. Example: "Day 1 Breakfast," "Day 1 Lunch," etc.
- Write the foods listed for that meal on the index card. Repeat this for all four days. On day 5, begin using day 1 again.

After the first week, the whole day's menu could be written on one larger index card and meals could be shuffled around for variety. Example: Day 1 Lunch served for Day 1 Dinner, Day 2 Breakfast served for Day 2 Lunch, etc.

You can create a shopping list on another index card for ease of picking up groceries in the supermarket since substitutions are not recommended.

Knowing You Are Getting Better

The journey back to health and vitality for those suffering from food intolerances begins with being able to evaluate your progress. Using a symptom checklist, you can see how well the diet and lifestyle changes are working. Completing a symptom checklist every 30–60 days can be a valuable tool for health-care providers who may offer suggestions for altering your regime. So mark your calendar and complete a symptom checklist like the one on this page regularly.

Symptom Checklist

Date _____

Symptom Point Scale: Use the point scale below to rate each symptom frequently associated with food intolerances.

0 = Never have symptom
1 = Occasionally have symptom but not severe
2 = Occasionally have severe symptom
3 = Frequently have symptom but not severe
4 = Frequently have severe symptom

Digestive Tract
Nausea and vomiting   _____
Diarrhea   _____
Constipation   _____
Bloated feeling   _____
Belching or passing gas   _____
Stomach pains or cramps   _____
Heartburn   _____
Blood and/or mucous in stools _____

                        Total _____

Joints and Muscles
Pains or aches in joints   _____
Arthritis   _____
Stiffness   _____
Pain or aches in muscles   _____
Feeling of weakness or tiredness _____

Swollen joints   _____

Pains in legs   _____

                     Total   _____

Head

Headaches   _____

Faintness   _____

Dizziness   _____

Insomnia, sleep disorder   _____

                     Total   _____

Mouth and Throat

Chronic coughing   _____

Gagging, frequently clearing throat   _____

Sore throat, hoarseness, loss of voice   _____

Swollen or discolored tongue, lips   _____

Canker sores   _____

Itching on roof of mouth   _____

                     Total   _____

Weight

Binge eating/drinking   _____

Craving certain foods   _____

Excessive weight gain   _____

Compulsive eating   _____

Fluid retention   _____

                     Total   _____

Eyes

Watery or itchy eyes   _____

Red, swollen, or sticky eyelids   _____

Bags or dark circles under eyes   _____

                     Total   _____

Nose

Stuffy nose   _____

Chronically red, inflamed nose   _____

Sinus problems   _____

Hay fever   _____

Sneezing attacks   _____

Excessive mucous   _____

                          Total   _____

Emotions

Mood swings   _____

Anxiety, fear, nervousness   _____

Anger, irritability, aggressiveness   _____

Argumentativeness   _____

Frustration; frequent crying   _____

Depression   _____

                          Total   _____

Mind

Poor memory   _____

Difficulty completing projects   _____

Underachiever   _____

Confusion   _____

Easily distracted   _____

Difficulty making decisions   _____

                          Total   _____

Lungs

Chest congestion   _____

Asthma, bronchitis   _____

Shortness of breath   _____

Persistent cough   _____

Wheezing   _____

                          Total   _____

Skin

Acne   _____

Itching   _____

Hives, rash, dry skin   _____

Hair loss   _____

                        Total   _____

Ears

Itchy ears   _____

Earaches, ear infections   _____

Ringing in ears   _____

Hearing loss   _____

                        Total   _____

Heart

Irregular or skipped heartbeat   _____

Rapid or pounding heart   _____

Chest pain   _____

                        Total   _____

Energy and Activity

Apathy, lethargy   _____

Fatigue   _____

Hyperactivity   _____

Restlessness   _____

Poor physical coordination   _____

Stuttering or stammering   _____

Slurred speech   _____

                        Total   _____

Other

Frequent illness	_____
Frequent or urgent urination	_____
Genital itch or discharge	_____
Anal itch	_____

Total _____

Grand Total _____

Circle those that have the highest score. See what scores differ each month and how the total score changes when you follow a food-allergy diet.

5

DIETS FOR TREATING FOOD ALLERGIES

The healthy intestine allows only nutrients to pass through the bloodstream. When the intestinal wall is damaged, undigested molecules of protein, fat, and starches can enter. These substances are recognized as foreign invaders and can trigger responses in the gut and other organs of the body. Thus, food may trigger symptoms of aching joints, itchy skin, fatigue, indigestion, headaches, and constipation.

Treatment approaches differ for food allergies versus food intolerances/sensitivities. Food allergy is usually treated with appropriate testing; then total avoidance of the substance is advised. Food intolerance has less defined symptoms and diagnosis. Minimizing exposure to common food allergens is a major factor in regaining health and vitality. For many, the four-day rotation diets will help reduce exposure to the same food allergens while promoting intestinal healing. A four-day rotation diet is usually followed for a minimum of 30–90 days. Some physicians even recommend following a four-day rotation diet for six months to a year. After the specified period, reactive foods are usually introduced gradually to see what reaction occurs. Some people can begin to eat some of their reactive foods on a limited basis.

About the Four-Day Rotation Diet

One of the most helpful ways of reducing food sensitivities or food intolerances is to follow a four-day food rotation diet. The purpose of this regimen is to minimize exposure to allergens in a food by consuming that food only once every fourth day.

Since the microvilli in the small intestine regenerate every three to four days, damage done by a particular food is limited to a one-day exposure and then the digestive tract heals itself before that food is eaten again.

Milk products, eggs, wheat, and corn are the major food intolerances but each person may have a totally unique list of reactive foods. One person's poison may provide another individual an excellent nutrition.

Highly sensitive people may even need to vary the type of vegetable oils used each day. Fortunately, many different kinds of vegetable oils are available—sunflower, sesame, olive, walnut, avocado, corn, safflower.

If you have symptoms during the four-day rotation period, write them down (i.e., "lots of gas during the day" or "heartburn after eating dinner"). Should these symptoms recur, certain foods may be causing a problem. Further elimination may be needed to identify which food is causing the symptoms.

After continuing on a rotation-diet regime for three to six months, you may begin to reintroduce foods and evaluate if they still cause problems. Each week introduce one new food and record any unusual symptoms—attitude change, alertness, aches and pains, rapid pulse, hearing or vision differences, fatigue, etc. Since many foods cause delayed reactions up to 72 hours after they are eaten, you need to be alert for symptoms up to three days after consuming it. If there is a reaction, continue to avoid that food. If there is no reaction, add that food to your rotation diet every four days. If you eat the food more frequently than that you may redevelop a sensitivity to that food.

Variety is the secret to living with food sensitivities. Avoid eating the same foods day after day. Experimenting with new flours and ingredients can be a rewarding experience in meal planning. New tastes and textures will delight the palate of many food-sensitive individuals.

A four-day rotation diet takes a high level of commitment and compliance. You'll need time, motivation, and family support to make this step in the treatment process a reality.

To begin, stop eating mixtures of food where hidden ingredients may be present, so that food tolerances can be carefully considered. Eating a plain and simple diet keeps food allergens to a minimum and allows for healthy intestinal recovery. A healthy gut results in improved nutritional status in the body.

One of the major problems in planning a rotation diet is to find a complete list of all foods within one food family. A complete guide to most foods is included in the Food Family Indexes in Appendix B.

Four-Day Rotation Diet Menus

Your four-day rotation diet plan must be individualized because no two people have the same food sensitivities. This process can seem like a monumental task for someone unfamiliar with food family groupings and little interest in planning meals. This book has done the work for you.

Wheat-Free Diet

Many processed foods contain wheat as an ingredient; therefore, it is important to know the names of ingredients that indicate the presence of wheat.

all-purpose flour
bran
bread crumbs
bread flour
bulgur
cake flour
cracked wheat flour
cracker meal and crumbs

durum
enriched flour
farina flour
gluten flour
graham crackers and crumbs
graham flour
hydrolyzed vegetable protein (HVP)**
malt†
malt syrup†
monosodium glutamate (MSG)**
pastry flour
phosphated flour
semolina
wheat
wheat flour
wheat germ

Wheat-Free Four-Day Rotation Diet

❧ Day 1

Breakfast	Oatmeal, Milk, Grapes
Lunch	Tuna salad, Rice Flour Muffins*, Fresh fruit cup
Dinner	Baked flounder, Rice, Asparagus, Cole slaw
Snacks	Oatmeal Cookies*

*Recipe included
**Gluten and/or wheat is often present but not always.
†Although gluten is not present in these products, the protein of malted barley may bring about a reaction to those sensitive to gluten.

⚽ *Day 2*

Breakfast	Amaranth Granola*, Apple
Lunch	Ground beef patty, French fries, Carrot salad
Dinner	Flank steak, Baked potato, Spinach, Tomato salad
Snacks	Apple Crisp*

⚽ *Day 3*

Breakfast	Teff Banana Muffins*, Papaya
Lunch	Italian Chicken*, Fresh fruit salad
Dinner	Cornish hen, Cornbread Stuffing*, Peas, Romaine lettuce
Snacks	Teff Chocolate Chip Cookies*

⚽ *Day 4*

Breakfast	Orange Quinoa Muffins*, Grapefruit
Lunch	Cheese pizza with Quinoa Pizza Crust*
Dinner	Lamb chop, Baked sweet potato, Green beans
Snacks	Strawberries, Orange Quinoa Muffins*

*Recipe included

Corn-Free Diet

Corn is one of the most widely used ingredients in America because it is easily and cheaply grown. Corn can be found in practically all processed foods and therefore is one of the most difficult foods to avoid. Learning how to identify corn in its many forms is the first step in developing a corn-free diet.

Corn can be made into corn syrup, cornmeal, corn oil, and cornstarch. It can be further processed into:

modified food starch**
dextrin
fructose
maltodextrins
dextrose
lactic acid
sorbitol
mannitol
caramel color
alcohol

Corn is used in the preparation of more foods than any other edible grain. Below is only a partial list of some of the many foods in which corn may be used.

baby foods
bacon
baking mixes
baking powders
batters for frying
beers
bleached wheat flours
bourbon and other whiskeys
breads and pastries
cakes

**Modified food starch can also be derived from other ingredients, such as tapioca, potatoes, or wheat.*

candles
carbonated beverages
catsups
cereals
cheeses
chili
chop suey
chow mein
coffee, instant
colas
cookies
confectioners' sugar
cream pies
eggnog
fish, prepared and processed
foods, fried
French dressing
frostings
fruits, canned and frozen
fruit juices
fruit pies
frying fats
gelatin desserts
glucose and fructose products
graham crackers
grape juice
gravies
grits
gums, chewing
gin
ginger ale
hams, cured
Harvard beets
ices
ice cream
jams and jellies

leavening agents and yeasts
liquors
margarine and shortenings
meats, processed and cold cuts
milk, in paper cartons
monosodium glutamate (MSG)
peanut butter and canned peanuts
pickles
powdered sugar
puddings and custards
salad dressings
salt
sandwich spreads
sauces for sundaes, meats, fish, etc.
sausages
sherbets
soft drinks
spaghetti
soups, creamed, thickened, and vegetable
soy milk
syrups, corn
teas, instant
tortillas
vanillin
vegetables, canned, creamed, and frozen
vinegar, distilled
waffles
wines

Remember to read the labels. Some of the products may be corn-free.

Corn can also be used in other ways. Plastic food wrappers, waxed paper cartons for milk and some juices, paper cups, and wax-coated paper plates are dusted with cornstarch to prevent sticking. Cornstarch is even in body powders, cosmetics, tooth-pastes, and soaps. Corn products are used in many medicines and vitamins. Corn may also be used as an adhesive for postage stamps and envelopes.

Because of the widespread use of corn, the only way to be sure to avoid it is by preparing all foods at home. Corn-free cooking is still the easiest part of staying on a corn-free diet. Simply substitute another starch for thickening foods. Buy corn-free baking powder and use maple syrup, honey, or sugar in place of corn syrup. Use corn-free oil, such as safflower oil.

Corn-Free Four-Day Rotation Diet

Day 1

Breakfast	Spelt Biscuits*, Strawberries
Lunch	Ground beef patty, French fries, Carrot salad
Dinner	Flank steak, Baked potato, Broccoli, Fresh fruit cup
Snacks	Spelt Chocolate Chip Cookies*

Day 2

Breakfast	Oatmeal, Milk, Banana
Lunch	Italian Chicken*, Oat Biscuits*, Fresh fruit salad
Dinner	Cornish hen, Oatmeal Shortbread*, Peas, Romaine lettuce
Snacks	Raisin Oatmeal Cake*

*Recipe included

≈≼   *Day 3*

Breakfast   Amaranth Granola*, Nut Milk*, Prunes
Lunch   Tuna salad, Amaranth Muffin*, Grapes
Dinner   Broiled salmon filet, Rice, Green beans
Snacks   Chocolate Pecan Amaranth Brownies*

≈≼   *Day 4*

Breakfast   Poached egg on whole wheat toast,
            Grapefruit
Lunch   Cheese pizza, Corn-free pizza crust
Dinner   Lamb chop, Baked sweet potato, Asparagus
Snacks   Ice cream**

Egg-Free Diet

Egg is probably the second most common food allergy in infants and young children, with egg whites causing the most problems.

Eggs are found in most processed foods. Sometimes the presence of eggs is not indicated on the label. For example, egg whites may be brushed on breads, rolls, pretzels, and other baked goods to give a glazed effect. Wine, beer, real root beer, coffee, bouillon, and consommé may be clarified with egg.

Egg is present if the label indicates any of the following:

albumen
ovalbumin
globulin
ovomucin

*Recipe included
**Corn-free

ovomucoid
powdered or dried egg
silicoalbuminate
vitellin
ovovitellin
yolk
livetin

Cooking Suggestions

For cake mixes, use 1 teaspoon of vinegar for each egg called for in the recipe. Since egg is a binder, baked goods made without eggs will crumble easily. It is best to make cupcakes instead of a full-size cake, and try one of the following.

- Use 1 teaspoon of xanthan gum in each recipe to help hold the baked good together.
- Add an extra half teaspoon of egg-free baking powder for each egg called for in a recipe.

For thickening cream dishes and sauces, add extra flour or cornstarch.

A good substitute for 1 egg in this kind of recipe is:

2 tablespoons allowed starch
½ tablespoon allowed shortening
½ teaspoon baking powder
2 tablespoons liquid such as water, juice, rice
    beverage, etc.

Grease and lightly flour the cookie sheet to prevent cookies from spreading.

Add extra ingredients like raisins, nuts, coconut, seeds, or spices to disguise the flavor of egg-free cookies and cakes.

Substitute mashed bananas, apricot puree, or pureed vegetables in place of eggs (2 tablespoons for each egg replaced).

Use unflavored gelatin (1 teaspoon dry gelatin mixed with 2 tablespoons liquid) to replace an egg.

Since homemade egg-free mayonnaise generally tastes more like flour and vinegar mixed together, it is best to avoid recipes calling for mayonnaise.

Egg-Free Four-Day Rotation Diet

Day 1

Breakfast	Teff Banana Muffins*, Grapefruit
Lunch	Tuna salad, Rice Flour Muffin*, Fresh fruit cup
Dinner	Baked flounder, Rice, Asparagus, Cole slaw
Snacks	Teff Chocolate Chip Cookies*

Day 2

Breakfast	Amaranth Granola*, Milk, Banana
Lunch	Cheese Pizza
Dinner	Lamb chop, Baked potato, Spinach, Tomato salad
Snacks	Apple Crisp*

Day 3

Breakfast	Spelt Biscuits*, Strawberries
Lunch	Italian Chicken, Spelt Bread*, Fresh fruit salad

*Recipe included

Dinner	Cornish hen, Cornbread Stuffing*, Peas, Romaine lettuce
Snacks	Quinoa Raisin Cookies*

❧ Day 4

Breakfast	Oatmeal, Nut Milk*, Prunes
Lunch	Ground beef patty, French fries, Carrot salad
Dinner	Flank steak, Baked sweet potato, Green beans
Snacks	Oatmeal Cookies*

Milk-Free Diet

Milk allergy is the most common allergy among infants and children under the age of three because of their immature or inefficient gastrointestinal systems. Milk allergy can cause a variety of symptoms throughout life. For example, after a period of avoidance and freedom from symptoms, the symptoms may change if milk is once again ingested. An infant may suffer from diarrhea, but when older, the young child may suffer from rhinitis (chronic stuffy nose).

Milk has many different protein fractions, but casein and whey are the most likely to cause reactions.

The whey fraction, which contains lactalbumin and β-lactoglobulin, causes the most reactions. Individuals who are allergic only to the whey (not the casein) may be able to tolerate goat's milk since the whey fraction differs from cow's milk, or they may tolerate powdered, boiled, or evaporated cow's milk,

*Recipe included

since the whey protein is changed by the heating process. Those allergic to the whey (lactose intolerant) will have to avoid cottage cheese and other soft processed cheeses but may be able to tolerate hard cheese, such as Swiss, Edam, Parmesan, cheddar, Gruyère, and Romano.

Casein remains stable during the heating process, so powdered, evaporated, or boiled milk cannot be consumed by a person who has a casein sensitivity. The casein is similar both in goat's milk and cow's milk, so both must be avoided. Even "nondairy" creamers, imitation processed cheese, imitation cream cheese, imitation sour cream, and soybean-based ice cream may contain casein.

Labels may have one of the following names if a product contains milk or milk protein:

lactose
caseinate
potassium caseinate
casein
lactalbumin
lactoglobulin
curds
wheys
milk solids

Goat's milk may be tolerated by some people who cannot tolerate cow's milk. The best way to assess tolerance is to try fresh goat's milk. If that does not produce symptoms, try canned evaporated goat's milk in recipes listing milk as an ingredient.

Substitutions for Milk in Recipes

An equal amount of any liquid can be substituted for milk.

Goat's milk, fresh, powdered, or evaporated, if tolerated
Soy milk; add 1 teaspoon vanilla or lime juice to improve
    the flavor
Banana, nut, or oat milk

Vegetable water, that is, water used to cook vegetables
  (add 1 tablespoon extra shortening to recipe)
Fruit juices or vegetable juices (add 1 tablespoon extra
  shortening or oil to recipe)
For sour cream, mix ½ cup allowed starch and ¾ cup
  water, soy milk, or goat's milk; stir in 2 tablespoons
  vinegar

Cooking Suggestions for Milk-Free Diet

Try fruits or fruit juices in place of milk on hot cereal.

Chill soy milk first and add flavoring such as
  vanilla extract.
Freeze fresh goat's milk first, then thaw; this eliminates
  some of the strong flavor and odor.
Use kosher margarine, bread, and processed meats
  that do *not* contain milk.
Use fruit juice in place of milk when making
  quick breads.
Use pure broth as a substitute for milk in sauces
  and gravies.
Fry foods in safflower oil or allowed oil instead of
  butter or margarine.

Milk-Free Four-Day Rotation Diet

❧ Day 1

Breakfast	Oatmeal, Nut Milk*, Grapefruit
Lunch	Sliced turkey on romaine lettuce, Oatmeal Muffin*, Carrots and celery, Grapes
Dinner	Broiled chicken, Baked sweet potato, Asparagus, Cole slaw
Snacks	Lemon Oatmeal Squares*

✒ *Day 2*

Breakfast	Corn flakes, Rice beverage, Banana
Lunch	Tuna salad, Rice Crackers*, Tomato and cucumbers
Dinner	Poached salmon, Rice, Green beans, Broiled tomato half
Snacks	Popcorn

✒ *Day 3*

Breakfast	Spelt Biscuit*, Nut butter, Orange juice
Lunch	Ground beef patty, Spelt Bread*, Lettuce and tomato, Fresh fruit salad
Dinner	Broiled beef steak, Baked potato, Carrots, Leaf lettuce salad
Snacks	Spelt Flour Plum Coffeecake*

✒ *Day 4*

Breakfast	Rice and Barley Muffins*, Scrambled egg, Strawberries
Lunch	Ham slice, Orange Barley Flour Bread*, Spinach salad, Apple
Dinner	Pork chop, Cornbread Stuffing*, Broccoli, Bibb lettuce salad
Snacks	Barley Banana Spice Bars*

*Recipe included

Gluten-Free Diet

The ingestion of even small amounts of gluten by gluten-intolerant individuals can lead to damage in the small intestine that may increase the risk of lymphoma. Celiac disease and dermatitis herpetiformis, a skin condition closely related to celiac disease, are the primary diseases treated with a gluten-free diet.

Present medical evidence suggests that eating foods with zero levels of gluten will enable these individuals to avoid serious long-term health risks.

Avoiding foods that may contain gluten can be a difficult task for someone who eats convenience foods frequently. Meal planning usually requires homemade soups or stews, fresh fruit and vegetables, rice crackers, potato chips, and unbreaded meat products.

A general rule of thumb is to eliminate these foods that are frequently made with wheat:

beer
biscuits
bologna
bouillon cubes
bread
cakes
cereals
chocolate candy
cocomalt
cooked meat dishes
cookies
cornbread
crackers
doughnuts
dumplings
flour

*Recipe included

flour-rolled meats
gluten bread
gravies
griddle cakes
ice cream
liverwurst
lunch ham
macaroni
matzos
muffins
pastries
rolls
scones

Gluten-Free Four-Day Rotation Diet

❧ Day 1

Breakfast	Grits, Scrambled egg, Orange juice
Lunch	Taco salad (ground beef), Corn chips
Dinner	Rib eye steak, Corn, Spinach, Tomato salad
Snacks	Popcorn, Orange wedges

❧ Day 2

Breakfast	Yogurt, Rice Bran Muffins*, Banana
Lunch	Tuna salad, Potato chips, Carrot salad
Dinner	Broiled salmon, Baked potato, Mixed vegetables, Cole slaw
Snacks	Rice Pudding*

∾ Day 3

Breakfast   Canadian Bacon, Corn Muffin*,
      Papaya Cubes

Lunch   Ham sandwich on Rice Flour Yeast
      Bread*, Leaf lettuce, Fresh fruit salad

Dinner   Pork chop, Baked sweet potato,
      Green beans, Leaf lettuce salad

Snacks   Ice cream**

∾ Day 4

Breakfast   Turkey Sausage, Rice Flour Muffin*, Apple

Lunch   Chef's salad (turkey and cheese),
      Romaine lettuce, Rice Crackers*

Dinner   Baked chicken, Rice, Broccoli,
      Cucumber salad

Snacks   Apple juice, Rice Flour Brownies*

Combination Allergen Menus

Avoiding a single food or food allergen may be difficult enough, but there are some people who need to avoid several common allergens and still get variety in their meals.

Every effort was made to keep these menus simple and tasty. The four-day regimen can be repeated and modified to meet individual preferences.

*Recipe included
**Wheat-free, gluten-free

Gluten-Free, Milk-Free, Egg-Free
Four-Day Menu

✤ Day 1

Breakfast	Ground Turkey Sausage, Grits, Grapefruit
Lunch	Chicken Caesar salad, Cornbread*
Dinner	Orange glazed Cornish hen, Cornbread Stuffing*, Broccoli, Fresh fruit salad
Snacks	Peanut Butter Cookies*

✤ Day 2

Breakfast	Steamed rice, Soy or Nut Milk*, Banana
Lunch	Ground beef patty, French fries, Cole slaw
Dinner	Broiled beef fillet, Baked potato, Asparagus, Tomato-and-cucumber salad
Snacks	Rice Flour Brownies*

✤ Day 3

Breakfast	Corn Muffins*, Strawberries
Lunch	Ham slices, Cornbread*, Carrot salad
Dinner	Pork tenderloin, Baked sweet potato, Green beans, Romaine lettuce salad
Snacks	Popcorn, Pear

*Recipe included

☙   *Day 4*

Breakfast	Rice Flour Muffin*, Papaya wedges
Lunch	Salmon salad, Rice crackers*, Waldorf salad
Dinner	Broiled grouper, Wild rice, Peas, Red leaf lettuce Salad
Snacks	Applesauce Raisin Cookies*

Wheat-Free, Egg-Free, Milk-Free Four-Day Menu

☙   *Day 1*

Breakfast	Grits, Orange juice
Lunch	Sliced turkey on romaine lettuce, Spicy Cornbread*, Orange wedges
Dinner	Baked chicken, Cornbread Stuffing*, Carrots
Snacks	Banana Cornmeal Spoonbread*

☙   *Day 2*

Breakfast	Oatmeal, Nut Milk*, Applesauce
Lunch	Ground beef patty, Oatmeal Biscuit*, Tomato salad, Apple

*Recipe included

Dinner	Broiled beef steak, Baked potato, Broccoli
Snacks	Raisin Oatmeal Cake*

❧ Day 3

Breakfast	Rice Flour Strawberry Muffins*, Banana
Lunch	Tuna on Red Leaf Lettuce, Quick Rice Bran Bread*
Dinner	Broiled salmon, Rice, Asparagus, Banana
Snacks	Puffed Rice Balls*

❧ Day 4

Breakfast	Canadian bacon, Rice-and-Barley Muffin*, Honeydew melon wedge
Lunch	Ham on Bibb lettuce, Orange Barley Flour Bread*
Dinner	Pork chop, Sweet potato, Cucumber salad, Melon balls
Snacks	Barley Flour Sugar Cookies*

Gluten-Free, Milk-Free Four-Day Menu

❧ Day 1

Breakfast	Canadian bacon, Rice bread, Strawberries
Lunch	Ham salad, Rice Crackers*, Tomato and cucumber salad, Plum

*Recipe included

Dinner	Pork chop, Savory Rice Dressing*, Carrots, Red leaf lettuce salad
Snacks	Rice Flour Lemon Squares*

ঌ৶ *Day 2*

Breakfast	Corn flakes, Rice beverage, Rice Flour Muffin*, Papaya cubes
Lunch	Ground beef patty, French fries, Cole slaw
Dinner	Flank steak, Acorn squash, Broccoli, Bibb lettuce salad
Snacks	Mini Fruitcake Cookies*

ঌ৶ *Day 3*

Breakfast	Scrambled egg, Grits, Orange wedges
Lunch	Ground turkey burger, Spicy Cornbread*, Carrot salad
Dinner	Roast turkey, Baked sweet potato, Green Beans, Fresh fruit salad
Snacks	Corn Muffin*, Grapefruit juice

ঌ৶ *Day 4*

Breakfast	Soy Rice Granola*, Nut Milk*, Banana
Lunch	Tuna rice casserole, Mixed vegetables, Waldorf salad

*Recipe included

Dinner	Broiled trout, Rice, Asparagus, Romaine lettuce salad
Snacks	Teff Applesauce Cake*

Wheat-Free, Corn-Free, Milk-Free Four-Day Menu

❧ Day 1

Breakfast	Scrambled egg, Millet muffin, Apple juice
Lunch	Chicken salad, Pumpkin millet bread, Cole slaw, Plum
Dinner	Cornish hen, Acorn squash, Broccoli, Cucumber salad
Snacks	Millet-Applesauce Cookies*

❧ Day 2

Breakfast	Cream of rice, Nut Milk*, Banana
Lunch	Tuna salad on Rice Flour Yeast Bread*
Dinner	Baked flounder, Rice, Spinach
Snacks	Rice Flour Muffin*

*Recipe included

&⁒ *Day 3*

Breakfast Amaranth Granola*, Papaya cubes

Lunch Ground beef patty, French fries,
Lettuce and tomato

Dinner Broiled flank steak, Baked potato,
Sliced tomato salad, Asparagus

Snacks Amaranth Cake*

&⁒ *Day 4*

Breakfast Orange Barley Flour Bread*, Orange juice

Lunch Turkey, Rice-and-Barley Muffin*, Orange

Dinner Lamb chop, Sweet Potato, Peas

Snacks Barley Flour Brownies*

Grain-Free, Egg-Free, Milk-Free Four-Day Menu

&⁒ *Day 1*

Breakfast Turkey sausage, Fried potatoes

Lunch Tuna salad on Lettuce, Potato chips

Dinner Broiled steak, Baked potato, Mixed greens,
Carrots

Snacks Potato chips

*Recipe included

❧ Day 2

Breakfast	Beef patty, Grapefruit, Sweet potato patty
Lunch	Taco salad with ground beef, lettuce, tomato
Dinner	Broiled salmon, Baked sweet potato, Green beans
Snacks	Sweet potato chips

❧ Day 3

Breakfast	Fresh pork bacon, Strawberries, Steamed pumpkin, Maple syrup
Lunch	Salmon, Caesar salad (no croutons)
Dinner	Venison Stew with Vegetables*
Snacks	Fresh fruit in Season

❧ Day 4

Breakfast	Venison cutlet, Pear, Mashed turnip patty
Lunch	Venison Stew with Vegetables*
Dinner	Broiled grouper, Mashed turnips, Spinach
Snacks	Banana

Fasting and Detox Diet

Those with severe digestion problems—frequently caused by using antibiotic drugs and over-the-counter pain medication—

*Recipe included

may find the fasting and detoxification diet the best way to jump-start their journey to digestive wellness.

A fast is frequently indicated in medical texts as the first step to correct severe digestive problems. In addition, each major religion in the world has a fasting ritual, which is often recommended for purifying the body. Fasting allows the digestive organs to rest, which aids in the loss of body fat and helps regulate liver detoxification.

A short two- to three-day fast can begin healing the intestinal wall and help control food sensitivities. Drinking lots of water (or fruit juice, if your body tolerates it) helps facilitate the elimination of toxins.

More restful sleep, heightened mental clarity, elimination of food cravings, and improved self-control have been reported following fasting and detoxification programs. Patrick Kingsley, M.D., recommends a five-day fast to ensure the adequate healing of the gastrointestinal mucosa. Any such fast should only be undertaken with the advice and monitoring of a qualified professional.

Jeffrey Bland, Ph.D., recommends a detoxification program using specific foods designed to provide extra nutrients to aid gastrointestinal healing. Many health-care practitioners are beginning to recommend high quality nonallergenic protein food along with nutrient supplements during detoxification to avoid the protein losses observed in animals who were put on similar fasting programs.

After a fast or detoxification regimen, you can add foods back slowly and note any signs of food sensitivity. Adding one new food every four days allows your best chance of assessing that food as a possible irritant.

Elimination Diet

An elimination diet is designed to include one food with a low antigen count from each food group. Be sure it's a food for which you have a strong tolerance. A low antigen menu for many is turkey, rice, green beans, pears, and safflower seed oil or avocado. Eat these foods exclusively for four days to assess the body symptoms—reduction in joint pains, headaches, mood swings, sleepiness, etc. If the symptoms persist, omit one food each day to identify the food creating the intolerance. Eat all you want of the nonreactive foods to satisfy your hunger.

Once the symptoms have disappeared, add one new food every four days to determine how well your body tolerates each food. Avoid any foods that cause your symptoms to reappear for a three- to six-month period before introducing them again. This regimen is not frequently followed as a treatment program because people tend to get bored and the time period needed to assess each food is so long. But if you can stick to it, this diet does pay off.

Desensitization

Desensitization is used both to diagnose and treat food allergies. The procedure involves placing a dose of the suspected allergen under the skin or under the tongue to provoke symptoms and determine what dose is needed to neutralize the symptoms. Some criticism of this technique has been made. The quality of the food-testing products has been questioned as food suppliers change and consistency of the testing solution throughout a year or over the years may decrease the effectiveness of this regime.

Desensitization does allow greater freedom of food choices and more varied menu selection—without the full range of symptoms—for many people who are unable to follow a strict rotation diet. An allergist can provide more details on this method of treatment for food allergies.

Food Combining

Various foods digest differently in the gastrointestinal tract according to some nutritional biochemists. Different foods require various times and enzymes for digestion. Certain combinations of foods may not be tolerated when eaten together so these are best avoided—especially if they cause gas or bloating. Melons and cucumbers are two common causes of digestive distress for some people.

Food combining is a concept of eating advocated by Herbert M. Shelton of the Dr. Shelton's Health School in San Antonio, Texas. This concept of eating evaluates all the factors that influence life—air, water, food, sunshine, rest, sleep, cleanliness, and emotional adjustment. Critics of food combining maintain that humans have eaten a complex varied diet throughout the ages based more on availability of foods than on correct combinations. But one of the features of this food plan is to create a structure for limiting food choices. Restricting foods chosen for a meal can limit calories and/or fat choices. It may even result in a greater variety of foods eaten than previously included in the diet. The more varied the diet, the less likely it is that food-sensitivity symptoms will occur.

Elimination Diet and Menus

An elimination diet is frequently recommended for people with severe food-allergy symptoms. The general purpose of the elimination diet is to help people stop consuming foods they may be intolerant to without using other testing procedures. The diet is milk-free, low fat, and gluten-free.

Elimination Diet Guidelines

- Drink two quarts of filtered water each day.
- Avoid coffee and foods that contain caffeine (tea, chocolate, soft drinks, even decaffeinated coffee).
- Eliminate pharmaceutical products that contain gliaden, such as Actifed, Advil, aspirin, Benadryl, Centrum, Excedrin, GasX, ibuprofen, Naprosyn, One-A-Day Multi-Vitamin, Pepcid, Premarin, Prednizone, Tagamet, and Tylenol (adapted from *Journal of Pediatric Gastroenterology Nutrition*, Vol. 19, No. 29, 1984).

- Eat only the allowed foods from the list that follows.
- Follow the diet for at least two to four weeks to assess your progress. An improvement is usually noted between 10 days and three weeks from the start of the diet. Add foods back very slowly—one per week—to identify which foods create symptoms.

Elimination Diet

Food Group	Allowed	Avoid
Meat, Fish, Poultry	Chicken, turkey, all legumes, dried peas and lentils, fish (salmon, halibut, flounder)	Beef, pork, lamb, cold cuts, frankfurter, sausage, processed meats, egg
Dairy Products	None	Milk, cheese, ice cream, cream, nondairy creamers
Starch/Bread/Cereals	White or sweet potato, rice, tapioca, corn-free and gluten-free products	All wheat, corn, rye, oats, millet, spelt, teff products
Vegetables	All vegetables, served plain, preferably fresh or frozen	Vegetables served creamed or in casseroles
Fruits	Unsweetened fresh, frozen, or water-packed, canned fruits	Fruit drinks, -ades, citrus, strawberries, dried fruit
Beverages	Unsweetened fruit or vegetable juices,	Milk, coffee, tea, cocoa, coffee

Food Group	Allowed	Avoid
Beverages	water, noncitrus herbal tea	substitutes such as Postum®, alcoholic beverages, soft drinks, sweetened beverages, citrus juices
Fats/Oils/Nuts	Cold/expeller pressed, unrefined, canola, flax, sunflower, sesame, pumpkin, squash seeds/ butters, salad dressings made from allowed ingredients, almonds, cashews, pecans, walnuts	Olive or sunflower oils, ghee (clarified butter), margarine, shortening, unclarified butter, refined oils, peanuts, salad dressings, and spreads

Elimination Diet Menu

❧ Day 1

Breakfast	Ground turkey patty, Cream of rice, Sliced banana
Lunch	Sliced turkey (not processed turkey lunch meat), Rice cakes, Lettuce and tomato, Applesauce
Dinner	Baked chicken, Brown rice, Green beans, Tossed salad with oil and vinegar
Snacks	Warm apple juice, Puffed rice cereal

Day 2

Breakfast	Rice flour waffle, Apple butter, Sliced peaches
Lunch	Chopped chicken, Tossed salad with oil and vinegar, Rice crackers, Banana
Dinner	Broiled salmon, Rice, Steamed carrots
Snacks	Fruit cup, Rice cakes

Day 3

Breakfast	Rice cakes, Cashew or almond butter, Pear
Lunch	Salmon strips on tossed salad with oil and vinegar, Rice cakes, Apple
Dinner	Baked snapper fillet, Baked potato, Asparagus
Snacks	Potato chips

Day 4

Breakfast	Steamed Rice, Fresh Fruit, Apple Juice
Lunch	Poached chicken, Stir-fried vegetables, Rice
Dinner	Sautéed flounder, Wild rice, Broccoli
Snacks	Popcorn

This menu is designed to be bland and use simple foods so that food allergens can be easily identified. During the first one to two weeks it is best to follow it closely without adding much seasoning to avoid introducing unsuspected allergens.

6

SPECIAL DIETS FOR SPECIAL NEEDS

Once you've discovered your food sensitivity, you must learn to avoid your problem food or additive. Here are some special diets for avoiding these common substances: sulfites, tartrazine, salicylate, MSG, lactose, yeast, and mold.

Sulfite-Free Diet

Sulfites are a major cause of food sensitivity due to a food additive. People with asthma are most affected by sulfites, but others can be sulfite sensitive as well. Some people with chronic urticaria or skin rash may be sensitive to sulfiting agents in foods.

Sulfites are widely used in the food supply and may not be listed on the ingredient label. Sulfites are used to control browning in foods, as a preservative in drugs and foods, and as a bleaching agent or dough modifier in breads. Some forms of sulfites that may be listed on the food label are: sodium sulfite, sodium metabisulfite, sodium bisulfite, sulfur dioxide, potassium sulfite, sodium sulfite, potassium metabisulfite, and potassium bisulfite.

Several foods and beverages are known for their high sulfite content. Dried apricots have the highest sulfite content of any food currently on the supermarket shelves. Wine has high quantities of sulfites because sulfur dioxide gas is used to sterilize wine barrels and sulfites are added to wine as a preservative.

Reactions to Sulfites

Asthmatic	Nonasthmatic
Flushing of skin	Skin rash
Dizziness	Loss of blood pressure
Reduced breathing	Itching skin
Wheezing	Diarrhea
Loss of consciousness	Dizziness
	Nausea
	Abdominal cramps
	Chest tightness
	Bloated, puffy hands or feet
	Tingling of skin

Foods Containing Sulfites

cereals containing dried apples, dried peaches, coconut
cookies, cakes, pastries with apricots, figs, or dried fruit
    (not prunes or dark raisins)
convenience potato products—mashed potatoes, scalloped
    potato dishes, frozen potatoes
grapes (sulfites used as a post-harvest fumigant to prevent
    rotting)
seafood products—shrimp, lobster, dried cod, scallops
mushrooms washed in sulfite solution
white grape juice, cider, beer, wine and wine coolers,
    apricot nectar, peach nectar
maraschino cherries
canned fruit fillings—apple, peach
dry salad dressing and gravy mixes plus dehydrated
    vegetable mixes (e.g., soup)
relishes, sauerkraut
wine vinegar, horseradish, pickles, olives

Beware of Salad Bars

Many reactions to sulfites have been attributed to salad bars. Sulfites are used on fresh fruits, guacamole, and lettuce to inhibit browning.

Restaurants have altered their use of sulfites on salad bar items but sensitive people would do best to *ask* before indulging.

Tartrazine-Free Diet

Food dyes, particularly tartrazine (FDA Yellow No. 5), are implicated as the cause of acute and chronic skin rashes or urticaria. Tartrazine is used in many foods, medications, and personal hygiene products. Manufacturers are not required to list tartrazine on the food label, so call to check if you are unsure of any product.

Foods That May Contain Tartrazine

penny candies, caramels, fruit chews, fruit drops,
    butterscotch squares, candy corn
Filled chocolate (not pure chocolate)
Soft drinks, fruit drinks, fizzy lemonade (except plain
    lemonade)
jellies
jams, marmalades (unless homemade)
stewed fruit sauces, fruit gelatins
fruit yogurt
ice cream, sherbet, ice milk
pie fillings
vanilla, butterscotch, or chocolate puddings
caramel custard (unless homemade)
whips and dessert sauces (vanilla custard)
commercial soups and soup mixes

commercially prepared cakes and frostings
cocoa, hot chocolate mixes
flavoring extracts—imitation banana and pineapple
orange drinks—Tang, Awake
Gatorade
gelatin desserts
Nondairy cream (liquid and powder)

Check with your pharmacist for information on drugs containing tartrazine.

Low-Salicylate Diet

Salicylates occur naturally in some foods—predominantly fruits. Other sources of acetylsalicylic acid are aspirin and aspirin-containing medications, methyl salicylate (salicin) or wintergreen/mint flavoring added to foods and personal-care products.

Salicylate-free diets are used in the treatment of chronic urticaria (hives). Many individuals who experience hives have a history of aspirin sensitivity.

Foods That Contain Salicylates

Fruits	Apricots, blackberries, boysenberries, cherries, currants, dewberries, gooseberries, huckleberries, maraschino cherries, melon, nectarines, peaches, raisins, raspberries, prunes, strawberries, cranberries, grapefruit, pineapples
Vegetables	Cucumbers, green bell peppers, alfalfa sprouts, asparagus, bean sprouts, broccoli, okra, parsnip, spinach, squash, sweet potatoes, zucchini, water chestnuts
Other Foods	Tea, root beer, beer, wine, vodka, cloves, pickles, catsup, Tabasco sauce, cider vinegar, wine vinegar, avocado, salad dressings

Foods to Eat on a Low-Salicylate Diet

Fruits	Apples, apple juice, bananas, figs, kiwi, lemon, mango, pear, pomegranate, red plums, rhubarb, seedless grapes
Vegetables	Cabbage, carrots, cauliflower, celery, corn, fresh tomatoes, green peas, lettuce, mushrooms, onions, turnips, white potatoes

MSG-*Free Diet*

MSG, also known as monosodium glutamate, is a flavor enhancer used in many foods. MSG is an amino acid produced by fermentation found in countless foods from soups and sauces to bouillon, and in more than 90 percent of prepared salad dressings. Nearly anything with the word *flavoring* on the label is likely to contain MSG.

It is estimated that over 25 percent of the population may be sensitive to MSG. This toxic food reaction can take many forms: headaches, migraines, nausea, rapid heartbeat, dizziness, asthma-like symptoms, and intestinal cramps.

MSG can cause brain cells to excite themselves to death. In some people, the slow deterioration is noted in years. Other people may experience brain cell hyperactivity more quickly, while some may never be affected. MSG is a food additive causing an excitotoxin effect at the brain receptor level. These excitotoxins eventually cause nerves to wear out just before they deteriorate from excessive stimulation.

If you suspect MSG is causing your symptoms, stop eating all processed foods. Eat only whole unprocessed foods for seven days. Then feast on your favorite foods that may contain any of these compounds and watch for symptoms.

These terms mean MSG is an ingredient:

autolyzed yeast
calcium caseinate

gelatin
glutamic acid
glutamine (flavor enhancer)
hydrolyzed protein
monopotassium glutamate (flavor enhancer)
monosodium glutamate (flavor enhancer)
sodium caseinate
textured protein
yeast extract
yeast nutrient

These may have forms of MSG:

baby food
barley malt
bouillon/broth/stock
carrageenan (seaweed extract breakdown catalyst)
enzymes
fermented
flavor(s)/flavoring(s)
malt extract
malt flavoring
maltodextrin
pectin (fruit extract for jelling)
protease enzymes
protease (enzyme/protein for jelling)
natural beef flavoring
natural chicken flavoring
natural flavor(s)/natural flavoring(s)
natural pork flavoring
protein fortified
protein modified
seasoning(s)
soy protein
soy protein concentrate
soy protein isolate
soy sauce

soy sauce extract
tuna fish
ultrapasteurized
whey protein
whey protein concentrate
whey protein isolate

Pay close attention to how you feel and any body symptoms that show up in the two days after you begin to eat processed foods again. Decide if eating these foods is worth continuing to have these symptoms.

Lactose-Free and Milk-Free Diets

Milk is one of the major causes of gastrointestinal problems in all age groups. Lactase, the intestinal enzyme needed for digestion of lactose, is usually present in adequate amounts during infancy unless an infection in the digestive tract occurs. A lactase deficiency can be quite common in adult African Americans, Asians, Native North Americans, and Eastern European Jews.

Symptoms of lactase deficiency include bloating, flatulence (gas), abdominal cramps, and diarrhea. Often these symptoms are called irritable bowel syndrome.

At birth, a normal infant has enough lactase to enable it to digest breast milk or a milk formula. This tolerance usually lasts until age four to five years when lactase levels begin to decrease. Some people discover that milk doesn't agree with them and consequently avoid it. Others keep testing to see how much milk, ice cream, and cheese they can digest.

To differentiate between the symptoms of lactose intolerance and milk-protein allergy, an allergy test is recommended. Milk protein hypersensitivity usually occurs within the first two or three months of life and disappears between the ages of two and four. Using a milk-free formula and milk-free diet is believed to alleviate the symptoms.

The menus and recipes in this book are milk-free. They can be used by people who are sensitive to milk protein and those who are sensitive to lactose.

People with lactase deficiency may choose to follow a low-lactose diet to minimize symptoms without giving up dairy products completely. Not all dairy foods have the same amount of lactose content. Hard cheeses (with the whey removed) contain limited amounts of lactose. Cottage cheese, yogurt, and ice cream have less lactose than milk does.

Lactose Content of Selected Dairy Products

	Amount	Lactose/Grams
Milk	1 cup	11
Buttermilk	1 cup	9–11
Whipped-cream topping	1 tablespoon	0.4
Light cream	1 tablespoon	0.6
Half & half	1 tablespoon	0.6
Low-fat yogurt	1 cup	11–15
Cheeses		
Blue	1 ounce	0.8
Cream	1 ounce	0.8
Parmesan	1 ounce	0.8
Colby	1 ounce	0.8
Camembert	1 ounce	0.1
Limburger	1 ounce	0.1
Cheddar	1 ounce	0.5
Gouda	1 ounce	0.5
American	1 ounce	0.5
Cottage cheese	1 cup	6.0
Butter	2 pats	0.1
Margarine	2 pats	0
Ice cream	1 cup	9
Sherbet, Orange	1 cup	4

Foods Containing Lactose

If you are lactose intolerant, you will probably find it best to eliminate most of the following foods from your diet until your symptoms are reduced. Then you can add a small portion of lactose-containing foods until you have identified your tolerance level.

Dairy foods	Milk, cheese, ice cream, sherbet made with milk, yogurt
Meats	Liverwurst, frankfurters, and cold cuts containing dry milk (all kosher meat products are milk-free)
Fruits and Vegetables	Any prepared with a cream sauce, whether fresh, frozen, or canned
Bread products	Any bread, cereal, pancakes, waffles, French toast made with milk
Miscellaneous	Candy, caramels, butterscotch, toffee; cakes, cookies, pies, puddings made with milk

Yeast-Free and Mold-Free Diet

Yeast-free and mold-free diets are recommended for those with yeast sensitivity and chronic yeast disorders of the gastrointestinal or urinary tract or genital area. Omitting these foods from the diet can minimize exposure to yeast allergens. To avoid mold in leftover foods, discard anything that is not eaten within two days.

These foods contain yeast and mold and should be minimized in the diet of those sensitive to yeast and molds:

- Baked goods made with yeast—breads, rolls, coffeecakes, pastries
- Wine, beer, whiskey, brandy, gin, rum, vodka, cider, ginger ale and root beer; fermented liquors from malt

- Foods that contain malt—malted milk drinks, cereals, candy. (Malt is sprouted grain that is dried.)
- Vinegar (distilled from grains, apple, or rice) and vinegar-containing foods—mayonnaise, salad dressings, mustard, catsup, Worcestershire sauce, barbeque sauce, chili sauce, shrimp sauce, pickles, relishes, green olives, sauerkraut, pickled vegetables, mincemeat, black tea, soy sauce
- Smoked and pickled meats and fish, including sausages, hot dogs, corned beef, pastrami, pickled tongue, bacon, ham
- Dried and candied fruits—raisins, apricots, dates, prunes, figs
- Fresh fruits with bruised and brown spots—peel and discard brown areas
- Fruit and vegetable juices unless freshly squeezed
- Melons, especially cantaloupe
- Peanuts and peanut butter due to aflatoxins
- Cheese (including cottage cheese and cream cheese), sour cream, buttermilk
- B vitamins unless stated yeast-free
- Antibiotics derived from molds—penicillin, streptomycin, tetracyclines

(Mold-sensitive individuals also report allergic symptoms around freshly cut grass, cereal grains, hay, and weeds, so avoid these as well.)

7

Main Dishes

Mexican Lasagna

(No Wheat, Egg, Gluten)

---

1 cup chicken, cooked, cut into
    bite-size pieces
1 small can enchilada sauce (mild/hot)
1 5-ounce can tomato sauce
9–12 6-inch corn tortillas
8 ounces shredded cheddar or
    mozzarella cheese

Preheat oven to 375° F. Combine chicken, enchilada sauce, and tomato sauce in a bowl. Lightly oil a 2-quart casserole dish and line bottom with 3–4 tortillas cut to fit. Spread with one-third of the chicken mixture. Sprinkle on one-fourth of the cheese. Layer another 3–4 tortillas on top. Spread with another one-third of the chicken mixture and sprinkle on another one-fourth of the cheese. Top with remaining tortillas, chicken mixture, and cheese. Bake uncovered about 40 minutes.

Makes 6 servings
One serving = 536   calories
             23 g   protein
             34 g   carbohydrates
             16 g   fat
       783 mg   sodium

Venison Stew with Vegetables

(No Wheat, Egg, Milk, Gluten)

1 pound venison, cut into bite-size pieces
1 cup chopped onion
2 garlic cloves, minced
4 carrots, cut into ½-inch pieces
2 stalks celery, cut into ½-inch pieces
2 large potatoes, cut into ½-inch pieces
2 cups water
1 teaspoon salt
½ teaspoon freshly ground black pepper

Brown venison in a non-stick pan. Add the remaining ingredients and simmer over medium heat 1–1½ hours until meat is tender.

Makes 4 servings
One serving = 291   calories
              23 g   protein
              16 g   carbohydrates
               5 g   fat
             303 mg sodium

✒

Chicken Salad

(No Wheat, Egg, Milk, Gluten)

---

salt
pepper
2 chicken breasts, split
4 red plums, pitted and diced
4 scallions (or green onions), sliced thin
16 pea pods
16 walnut halves

Lightly salt and pepper chicken breasts, then sauté them over medium heat about 4 minutes on each side until no longer pink. Remove from heat and let cool. Slice into bite-size pieces. Combine chicken with the remaining ingredients. Chill and serve with Walnut Oil Dressing. (See Index.)

Makes 2 servings
One serving = 297   calories
            26 g   protein
            12 g   carbohydrates
             9 g   fat
            18 mg   sodium

Black Bean Tortilla Casserole

(No Wheat, Gluten, Egg)

2 cups coarsely chopped onion
2 cloves garlic, minced
1 cup coarsely chopped green bell pepper
1 cup coarsely chopped red bell pepper
¾ cup picante sauce
1½ teaspoons ground cumin
2 15-ounce cans black beans, drained
1 14½-ounce can stewed tomatoes, undrained
   and chopped
12 6-inch corn tortillas
1½ cups shredded Monterey Jack cheese
1 cup shredded iceberg lettuce
½ cup seeded, chopped, unpeeled tomato
4 tablespoons sour cream

Place large nonstick skillet over medium heat until hot. Add onion and garlic, and sauté 4 minutes or until tender. Add bell peppers, and sauté 3 minutes or until tender. Add picante sauce, cumin, and black beans. Cook 5 minutes, stirring occasionally. Remove from heat, and set aside.

Preheat oven to 350°F. Coat a 13″ × 9″ × 2″ baking dish with vegetable oil. Spoon 1 cup of bean mixture into baking dish. Arrange 6 tortillas in a single layer over bean mixture; top with ½ of the cheese. Spoon 2½ cups of bean mixture over cheese. Arrange 6 remaining tortillas over cheese; top with remaining bean mixture.

Cover and bake 30 minutes. Uncover and top with remaining cheese. Bake, uncovered, another 5 minutes, or until cheese melts. Let stand 5 minutes before serving. Top with lettuce and tomato. Cut into 4½-inch squares; top each serving with 2 teaspoons sour cream.

Makes 6 servings
One serving = 496   calories
             18 g   protein
         269 g   carbohydrates
           8 g   fat
     703 mg   sodium

✦

Mushroom Barley Casserole

(No Wheat, Milk, Egg)

4 cups beef broth
¼ cup vegetable oil
2 tablespoons dried chopped onions
1 2½-ounce can mushroom pieces
1 cup pearl barley
1 teaspoon salt

Preheat oven to 350°F. Combine all ingredients in ungreased 2-quart casserole dish. Bake, uncovered, for 1 hour, stirring several times. Cover and bake 30 additional minutes.

Makes 8 servings
One serving = 126   calories
                3 g   protein
               18 g   carbohydrates
                5 g   fat
             299 mg   sodium

❧

Italian Chicken

(No Wheat, Egg)

---

2 chicken breasts, split
¼ cup barley flour
2 tablespoons grated Parmesan cheese
¼ teaspoon dried oregano leaves
¼ teaspoon dried basil leaves
¼ teaspoon salt

Preheat oven to 350°F. Wash chicken pieces and pat dry. Stir together flour, cheese, and herbs in a small bowl. Roll chicken in herb blend. Place chicken on a baking sheet. Bake until brown and tender, about 35–40 minutes.

Makes 4 servings
One serving = 197 calories
17 g protein
7 g carbohydrates
3 g fat
201 mg sodium

Crispy Fried Chicken

(No Wheat, Egg, Milk, Gluten)

½ cup brown rice flour
½ teaspoon salt
¼ teaspoon garlic powder
¼ teaspoon freshly ground black pepper
3 pounds broiler-fryer chicken
2 tablespoons vegetable oil

Preheat oven to 325°F. Combine rice flour, salt, garlic powder, and pepper in a paper bag; shake thoroughly. Shake chicken pieces, one at a time, in bag. In a medium skillet, brown chicken in oil until golden brown on all sides. Put chicken pieces on lightly oiled cookie sheet and bake 40 minutes.

Makes 4 servings
One serving = 348 calories
25 g protein
17 g carbohydrates
11 g fat
247 mg sodium

❧

Curried Chicken Casserole

(No Wheat, Egg, Milk, Gluten)

¼ cup chopped onion
1 small clove garlic, minced
½ cup chopped celery
1 teaspoon vegetable oil
½ teaspoon curry powder
¼ teaspoon white pepper
½ teaspoon caraway seeds
2 cups cooked diced chicken
2 cups cooked brown rice

Sauté onion, garlic, and celery in oil in a large frying pan. Add curry powder, pepper, and caraway seeds. Cook over very low heat 10 minutes. Add chicken and rice. Heat thoroughly and serve.

Makes 4 servings
One serving = 382 calories
23 g protein
34 g carbohydrates
2 g fat
211 mg sodium

✺

Potato Chip Baked Chicken

(No Wheat, Milk, Egg, Gluten)

---

3 pounds cut-up chicken pieces
¼ cup vegetable oil
1 cup finely crushed potato chips

Preheat oven to 400°F. Dip chicken in oil. Drain on paper towels. Roll the chicken in crushed chips. Arrange in greased, shallow baking dish. Cover tightly with foil. Bake 45 minutes until tender. Uncover the dish and continue to bake at least 15 minutes to brown chicken.

Makes 4 servings
One serving = 420   calories
              22 g protein
              17 g carbohydrates
              13 g fat
             497 mg sodium

⊲⅍

Chicken Casserole

(No Wheat, Egg, Milk, Gluten)

---

2 cups cooked diced chicken
1 cup chopped celery
2 tablespoons grated onion
2 tablespoons lemon juice
½ teaspoon salt
½ cup slivered almonds
1 cup crushed rice cereal

Preheat oven to 350°F. Combine all ingrédients, except rice cereal. Toss lightly. Pour into lightly greased 1½-quart casserole dish. Sprinkle with rice cereal. Bake 30 minutes until bubbly.

Makes 4 servings (Mixture can also be used as stuffing in green peppers or tomatoes.)
One serving = 287   calories
27 g   protein
10 g   carbohydrates
8 g   fat
397 mg   sodium

Beef and Rice Pizza

(No Wheat, Egg, Milk, Gluten)

1 pound ground beef
2 cloves garlic, minced
¼ teaspoon salt
1 tablespoon oregano
1 cup cooked brown rice
1 cup tomato puree
1 green pepper, sliced

Preheat oven to 350°F. Sauté ground beef with garlic, salt, and oregano. Pour off any fat as it cooks. Press rice into lightly oiled 9-inch pie pan. Pour ground beef mixture on top. Add tomato puree and green pepper slices. Bake 15–20 minutes.

Makes 4 servings
One serving = 396   calories
            29 g   protein
            31 g   carbohydrates
             3 g   fat
          306 mg   sodium

꿎

Ground Beef Sausage Patty

(No Wheat, Egg, Milk, Gluten)

½ pound lean ground beef
¼ teaspoon salt
1 teaspoon dried thyme
1 teaspoon dried oregano
½ teaspoon dried sage
½ teaspoon dried ginger

Mix ingredients together thoroughly. Refrigerate overnight for maximum flavor. Form into 8 meat patties. Sauté in skillet 5 to 7 minutes over medium heat. Turn. Cook 2 to 3 minutes longer, until done.

Makes 4 servings
One serving = 84   calories
                6 g protein
                2 g carbohydrates
                2 g fat
              108 mg sodium

Mexican Tortilla Pie

(No Wheat, Egg, Gluten)

1 teaspoon vegetable oil
1 clove garlic, minced
1/2 cup chopped onion
1/4 cup chopped green pepper
1 14 1/2-ounce can whole peeled tomatoes
1 4-ounce can chopped green chili peppers
1/4 cup tomato paste
2 teaspoons chili powder
1 1/2 teaspoons dried oregano
1/2 teaspoon ground cumin
1/4 teaspoon ground cayenne pepper
1/2 pound lean ground beef
8 large corn tortillas
4 ounces shredded low-fat mozzarella cheese

Preheat oven to 350°F. Combine oil, garlic, onion, and green pepper in skillet. Sauté over medium heat 5 minutes until onion is tender. Add tomatoes, chili peppers, tomato paste, chili powder, oregano, cumin, and cayenne pepper. In a separate skillet, brown beef until done, drain off any fat, and add to tomato mixture. Lightly oil a 9-inch pie pan and line with 4 tortillas. Pour half the meat-and-tomato mixture over tortillas. Sprinkle with half of the cheese. Layer the 4 remaining tortillas over mixture. Spread on the remaining meat mixture. Top with the remaining cheese.

Bake 20–25 minutes, or until cheese melts and tortillas are browned at the edges. Let stand 10 minutes before cutting into wedges.

Makes 4 servings
One serving = 317   calories
            15 g   protein
            24 g   carbohydrates
             3 g   fat
          403 mg   sodium

Rice Salmon Casserole

(No Wheat, Egg, Milk, Gluten)

1 tablespoon vegetable oil
1 medium onion, chopped
1 clove garlic, chopped
1 cup chopped celery
2 carrots, sliced
1 broccoli stalk, chopped
1 teaspoon caraway seeds
1/4 teaspoon celery seeds
1/2 teaspoon dried parsley
7 ounces canned salmon
1 cup cooked brown rice

Combine oil, onion, and garlic in a skillet over medium heat. Sauté until onion and garlic are translucent. Add celery, carrots, and broccoli. Sauté, stirring occasionally, until vegetables become bright and crisp—about 5 minutes. Stir in herbs, salmon, and brown rice. Toss gently and pour into serving dish or heat over low temperature in skillet until vegetables are tender. Serve hot with fruit salad.

Makes 2 servings
One serving = 328   calories
             26 g   protein
             22 g   carbohydrates
             9 g   fat
        406 mg   sodium

≈✦

Tuna and Rice Casserole

(No Wheat, Egg, Milk, Gluten)

---

1 6½-ounce can water-packed tuna, flaked
1½ cups cooked rice
¼ cup water
½ cup chopped fresh mushrooms
¼ cup chopped celery, tomato, or
    green pepper
¼ teaspoon dried basil or dill weed
Freshly ground black pepper to taste

Preheat oven to 375°F. Combine ingredients. Place in shallow baking dish. Bake, uncovered, until browned, about 20–25 minutes.

Makes 2 servings
One serving = 331   calories
           23 g   protein
           36 g   carbohydrates
            2 g   fat
    297 mg   sodium

❧

Zucchini Lasagna

(No Wheat, Egg, Gluten)

---

2 large zucchini, sliced ⅛- to ¼-inch thick
¼ cup cornstarch
2 cups spaghetti sauce
1 cup ricotta cheese
2 medium carrots, grated
½ cup grated Parmesan cheese

Preheat oven to 350°F. In a medium saucepan fitted with a steamer, steam zucchini slices 3 to 5 minutes to reduce some of the water content. Coat with cornstarch. Line bottom of casserole dish with layer of zucchini slices. Add about ¾ cup spaghetti sauce. Spread ½ cup ricotta cheese over mixture. Sprinkle with ½ of the carrots. Add another layer of zucchini slices, then another ¾ cup sauce, and rest of ricotta cheese and carrots. Add remaining zucchini slices. Spread the rest of the sauce and top with cheese. Bake 40–50 minutes.

Makes 4 servings
One serving = 230   calories
            13 g   protein
            14 g   carbohydrates
             6 g   fat
           516 mg sodium

҂

Savory Meatloaf

(No Wheat, Egg, Milk, Gluten)

———————

1 pound ground beef
½ teaspoon salt
3 tablespoons prepared minute tapioca or
* ½ cup cooked rice*
⅛ teaspoon freshly ground black pepper
1 6-ounce can tomato paste
¼ cup finely chopped onion
½ teaspoon salt
⅛ teaspoon dried sage

Preheat oven to 325°F. Combine all ingredients and mix well. Spoon into a 9″ × 5″ loaf pan. Press lightly. Bake 1 hour.

Makes 6 servings
One serving = 251   calories
           15 g   protein
           16 g   carbohydrates
            8 g   fat
          203 mg   sodium

Beef Stew

(No Wheat, Egg, Milk, Gluten)

---

1 pound beef, lamb, or veal cut for stew
1 celery stalk, cut in 1/2-inch pieces
1/2 medium onion, chopped
2 medium carrots, halved and cut into 1-inch
*   thick pieces*
3 tablespoons tapioca
1 teaspoon salt
1/2 teaspoon pepper
1 cup water
1 bay leaf

Preheat oven to 300°F. Combine all ingredients in Dutch oven or 2-quart casserole dish. Cover and bake 2½ hours. Remove bay leaf.

Makes 4 servings
One serving = 345   calories
             23 g   protein
             18 g   carbohydrates
             11 g   fat
            387 mg sodium

❧

Beef and Vegetable Pie

(No Wheat, Egg, Milk, Gluten)

---

1 pound ground beef
⅓ cup chopped onion
1 cup puffed rice cereal
2 tablespoons tomato puree, tomato sauce, or
*   catsup*
½ teaspoon salt
Dash of freshly ground black pepper
1 tablespoon margarine or vegetable oil
1½ cups coarsely chopped mixed fresh
*   vegetables (celery, green pepper, carrot*
*   slices, broccoli, asparagus pieces,*
*   green beans)*
½ cup diced mushrooms

Preheat oven to 400°F. Combine ground meat, onion, ¾ cup puffed rice cereal, tomato puree, salt, and pepper. Press mixture into bottom and sides of 9-inch pie plate. Bake 15 minutes. Drain off any fat and set pan shell aside. Reduce oven temperature to 350°F. Sauté vegetables in margarine or vegetable oil. Remove from heat and pour on top of meat. Add mushrooms and reserved ¼ cup puffed rice cereal. Bake 10 minutes more.

Makes 4 servings
One serving = 461 calories
              27 g protein
              22 g carbohydrates
              12 g fat
             341 mg sodium

Lebanese Meatballs

(No Wheat, Milk, Gluten)

½ pound ground beef
½ pound ground lamb
2 cloves garlic, crushed
½ cup chopped onion
⅓ cup chopped pine nuts
¼ cup chopped fresh parsley
½ teaspoon salt
1 teaspoon dried thyme
½ teaspoon curry powder
¼ teaspoon pepper
1 egg
2 tablespoons vegetable oil

Combine beef, lamb, garlic, onion, pine nuts, parsley, seasonings, and egg in a bowl. Mix until well blended. Shape into 12 1-inch balls. Heat vegetable oil in a large skillet over medium heat. Add the meatballs and cook for 10 minutes or until desired doneness is reached. Serve with rice.

Makes 4 servings
One serving = 357   calories
          21 g   protein
           7 g   carbohydrates
         12 g   fat
     348 mg   sodium

≈⅊

Eggplant Lasagna Casserole

(No Wheat, Egg, Gluten)

———————

1 *pound ground turkey or chicken*
½ *cup chopped onion*
¼ *cup chopped green pepper*
1 *clove garlic, minced*
1 *8-ounce can tomato sauce*
½ *teaspoon salt*
1 *teaspoon dried oregano leaves*
½ *teaspoon dried basil leaves*
½ *teaspoon dried marjoram leaves*
¼ *teaspoon freshly ground black pepper*
1 *pound eggplant, peeled and cut into ¼-inch*
    thick slices
1 *cup low-fat cottage cheese*
4 *ounces sliced low-fat mozzarella cheese*

Preheat oven to 350°F. In a medium skillet over medium heat, sauté ground turkey, onion, green pepper, and garlic. Stir in tomato sauce, salt, oregano, basil, marjoram, and pepper. Bring to boil, then reduce heat to simmer for 10 minutes. Remove from heat and set aside. Cook eggplant in boiling water just until tender, 2–3 minutes. Drain. Arrange eggplant slices in bottom of a large oiled baking dish. Spread on half the meat mixture. Spoon on cottage cheese. Top with the remaining eggplant slices and meat mixture. Lay mozzarella cheese slices on top. Bake 40–45 minutes. Let stand 5 minutes before serving.

Makes 4 servings
One serving = 288   calories
           23 g   protein
            8 g   carbohydrates
           11 g   fat
      618 mg   sodium

Crepes

(No Wheat, Gluten)

2 eggs
¼ cup milk
¼ cup water
½ cup brown rice flour
1 tablespoon sugar
1 tablespoon potato flour
1 tablespoon melted butter or vegetable oil

Combine all ingredients in blender, food processor, or mixer. Blend until smooth. Let batter stand at room temperature 15–20 minutes. Pour batter onto hot oiled griddle, just enough to coat bottom. After about 15–20 seconds, loosen edges of crepe and lift to see if bottom is browned. When browned, turn the crepe quickly. Cook for another 10–15 seconds. Slide onto warmed plate. Continue making crepes; be sure to oil the pan well between each one.

Makes 12 servings.

Dessert Crepes Fill each crepe with fruit. Roll up. Serve warm with yogurt or sour cream.

CREPES SUZETTE

½ cup butter
¼ cup powdered sugar
1 tablespoon grated orange peel
¼ cup orange juice
2 tablespoons brandy flavoring

Cream together butter and powdered sugar. Add grated orange peel, orange juice, and brandy flavoring. When ready to serve, put butter mixture in chafing dish or electric skillet. Heat until it bubbles. Using fork, dip each crepe into mixture, fold into quarters, and place on side of chafing dish. When all crepes are dipped, sprinkle with powdered sugar and serve.

Cheese Blintze Place tablespoon cottage cheese or bakers cheese in center of each crepe. Roll up. Place in chafing dish or warm serving dish. Top with yogurt or sour cream and dash of nutmeg or cinnamon.

One serving = 42 calories
2 g protein
8 g carbohydrates
2 g fat
27 mg sodium

❧

Vegetarian Shepherd's Pie

(No Wheat, Egg, Gluten)

MASHED POTATOES

> 8 potatoes, peeled and cut into small cubes
> ½ teaspoon salt
> 1 tablespoon butter or margarine

Cook potatoes in enough water to cover. Add salt. Bring to boil, then simmer till tender. Drain. Add butter. Mash. Milk or cream may be added (if tolerated). Set aside while you prepare the pie.

PIE

> ½ cup butter or margarine
> 1 medium onion, chopped fine
> 1 cup finely chopped celery
> 1 cup thinly sliced carrots
> 8 cups dry rice bread cubes
> 2 teaspoons ground sage
> ½ teaspoon dried marjoram leaves
> ½ teaspoon dried thyme leaves
> ½ teaspoon celery seeds
> ½ teaspoon salt
> 2 tablespoons minced fresh parsley
> 1½ cups water

Preheat the oven to 375°F. Prepare vegetable pie by sautéing butter, onion, celery, and carrots in skillet until celery is tender. Stir in bread cubes, sage, marjoram, thyme, celery seeds, salt, parsley, and water. Pour into oiled casserole dish. Top with the mashed potatoes. Bake 30–40 minutes, or until mashed potatoes are golden.

Makes 4 servings
One serving = 364 calories
8 g protein
42 g carbohydrates
14 g fat
386 mg sodium

Baked Polenta with Hazelnuts and Prunes

(No Wheat, Milk, Gluten)

---

2 cups tomato sauce
1 teaspoon ground cinnamon
1 cup packed, coarsely chopped pitted prunes
2 cloves garlic, minced
2 tablespoons fresh chopped parsley
½ cup hazelnuts
1 cup cornmeal or ½ cup cornmeal and
    ½ cup corn flour (not cornstarch)
1 cup cold water
2 cups boiling water
½ teaspoon salt
¼ teaspoon freshly ground black pepper
½ teaspoon grated nutmeg
2 tablespoons margarine or ghee
2 large eggs, beaten
1 tablespoon olive oil

Preheat oven to 350°F. Place the tomato sauce in a pan and add the cinnamon, prunes, garlic, and parsley. Cook together for 10 minutes over medium-low heat. Remove pan from heat and set aside.

Spread hazelnuts in a cake pan and toast in the oven for 12–15 minutes or until aromatic and lightly golden. Pour warm hazelnuts into a clean dish towel and wrap up. Rub the nuts together through the towel to remove the skins. Discard the skins. Chop the nuts and set them aside. Raise the oven temperature to 400°F.

Place the cornmeal in a large bowl. Add the cold water and mix well. Pour the boiling water over the mixture, whisking until it is smooth. (This technique prevents lumps from forming.) Transfer the mixture to a heavy pan. Add salt, pepper, and nutmeg. Slowly bring the mixture to a boil over medium heat, whisking constantly. When it is boiling, lower the heat and cook, stirring frequently with a spoon, until the polenta mixture is thick enough so that the spoon will stand up in it. When it is thickened, remove the pan from the heat. Add the butter and mix until it melts. Let the polenta cool slightly.

Lightly oil a 9" × 13" baking dish. Add the beaten eggs to the polenta, mixing constantly until they are incorporated. Pour half over the polenta into the baking dish. Spread half the tomato-prune sauce over the polenta in an even layer. Pour and spread remaining polenta over the sauce. Pour remaining sauce over the polenta layer. Sprinkle with the hazelnuts. Bake the polenta until it is bubbly, about 20–30 minutes. When cooked, remove it from the oven and let it settle for about 10 minutes before serving.

Makes 6 servings
One serving = 367 calories
6 g protein
48 g carbohydrates
18 g fat
412 mg sodium

꧁

Mediterranean Rice Salad

(No Wheat, Egg, Milk, Gluten)

---

1 cup uncooked brown or basmati rice
2 tablespoons olive oil
2 cups sliced zucchini (¼-inch slices)
1 teaspoon dried basil
1 teaspoon dried oregano
4 cups red leaf or romaine lettuce
2 cups fresh chopped spinach leaves
½ cup sliced black olives
⅓ cup oil-and-vinegar type salad dressing

Place rice and 2 cups water in a medium saucepan. Add 1 table-spoon olive oil to water. Bring to boil, then lower the heat and simmer rice, covered, until all the water has been absorbed and the rice is tender—about 25–30 minutes depending on type of rice used. Set rice aside. Combine 1 tablespoon olive oil and zucchini in skillet. Add basil and oregano. Sauté until zucchini is slightly browned. Break lettuce into bite-size pieces and toss with spinach leaves. Add rice, zucchini, olives, and salad dressing. Toss well. Serve immediately.

Makes 2 large servings
One serving = 347   calories
                    11 g   protein
                    38 g   carbohydrates
                    16 g   fat
                  306 mg   sodium

8

ACCOMPANIMENTS

Walnut Oil Dressing

(No Wheat, Egg, Milk, Gluten)

¼ cup walnut oil
¼ cup lemon juice
1 teaspoon dried crumbled rosemary or thyme
1 tablespoon finely chopped green pepper
½ teaspoon salt

Combine all ingredients in a bottle with a lid. Shake thoroughly.
Let stand at room temperature several hours. Shake again.

Makes ½ cup
One serving = 41   calories
           1 g   protein
           1 g   carbohydrates
           6 g   fat
     24 mg   sodium

Rice Flour Noodles

(No Wheat, Milk, Gluten)

2 eggs
2 teaspoons water
1 teaspoon salt
¼ cup cornstarch
1 cup rice flour

Using a fork or a whisk, beat eggs and water until frothy. Add remaining ingredients. Dough must be stiff but workable. Add more water or flour if necessary. Knead dough thoroughly on rice-floured board. Roll out dough as thin as possible. Cut into ¼-inch-wide strips. Let dry undisturbed at least 1 hour before cooking. Noodles will break easily if not allowed to dry. Cook in boiling salted water or broth for 10 minutes. May be served with spaghetti sauce.

Makes 2 cups dry noodles.
One serving (½ cup dry noodles) = 118   calories
4 g   protein
20 g   carbohydrates
2 g   fat
297 mg   sodium

~~❧~~

Savory Rice Dressing

(No Wheat, Egg, Milk, Gluten)

---

1 cup cooked brown rice
2 teaspoons vegetable oil
½ cup diced celery
¼ cup chopped onion
1 tablespoon dried parsley
¼ teaspoon salt
¼ teaspoon ground sage
1 cup sliced fresh mushrooms
1 cup chicken broth or tomato juice

Preheat oven to 325°F. In a medium pan over medium-low heat, sauté rice in vegetable oil until lightly browned. Add celery, onion, parsley, salt, sage, and mushrooms. Sauté 2 minutes longer. Add chicken broth and mix in to moisten rice. Cover and heat 15 minutes on medium heat or pour into casserole dish and bake 30 minutes.

Makes 4 servings
One serving = 119   calories
2 g   protein
19 g   carbohydrates
4 g   fat
208 mg   sodium

Cornbread Stuffing

(No Wheat, Milk, Egg, Gluten)

1 double batch Cornbread (See Index.)
1½ cups chopped onion
1½ cups chopped celery and celery leaves
½ cup vegetable oil or milk-free margarine
1 tablespoon salt
½ teaspoon freshly ground black pepper
1 tablespoon poultry seasoning
1 cup water or turkey or chicken broth

Preheat the oven to 200°F. Break the cornbread into fine crumbs and place on a baking sheet. Dry crumbs out for about 30 minutes in the oven. Sauté onion and celery in vegetable oil. Add seasonings and liquid. Pour over crumbs and mix until moistened. Stuff turkey and bake immediately, or bake separately in a 2-quart, greased casserole dish in a 350°F oven.

Makes enough to stuff one 12-pound turkey.
One serving of ½ cup = 136   calories
3 g   protein
21 g   carbohydrates
4 g   fat
291 mg   sodium

‹✍

Potato Soup

(No Wheat, Milk, Egg, Gluten)

⅓ *cup chopped onion or leek*
1 tablespoon olive oil
1 large baked potato
1 cup water or Nut Milk (See Index.)
½ *teaspoon freshly ground caraway*

In a small pan over medium heat, sauté the onion in oil until soft but not brown. Coarsely chop the baked potato in a food processor or blender. Add the remaining ingredients. Add more water if needed for desired consistency. Place all ingredients in a medium saucepan over low heat and simmer 5 minutes to heat and blend flavors.

Makes 2 servings
One serving = 107 calories
2 g protein
21 g carbohydrates
6 g fat
63 mg sodium

Onion Sauce

(No Wheat, Milk, Egg, Gluten)

---

1 or 2 large sweet onions, sliced thin
¼ cup water
Salt to taste
2–4 teaspoons olive oil

Pile the onions in a large frying pan or Dutch oven. Add the water. Cover tightly and steam over low heat for 15–20 minutes until quite soft. Pour the onion mixture into a food processor or blender and puree. Season with salt and olive oil. Use to sauce vegetables, meat, fish, or poultry. Excellent on new potatoes and green peas.

Makes 2 servings
One serving = 52   calories
           0 g   protein
           4 g   carbohydrates
           5 g   fat
      37 mg   sodium

ᗕ৶

White Sauce

(No Wheat, Egg, Milk, Gluten)

---

2 tablespoons vegetable oil
1 tablespoon tapioca or cornstarch
½ teaspoon salt
⅛ teaspoon white pepper
1 cup plain soy milk

Put vegetable oil in saucepan. Stir in tapioca or cornstarch, salt, and pepper. Remove from heat. Gradually add milk, and mix until smooth. Return to medium heat and bring to boil, stirring constantly. Boil 1 minute.

Makes ¾ cup sauce
One serving of 2 tablespoons = 94 calories
1 g protein
11 g carbohydrates
8 g fat
119 mg sodium

This recipe can also be used as Almond Sauce by adding 2 tablespoons toasted finely chopped, blanched almonds; serve with fish or vegetables.

For cheese sauce, add ¼ cup finely shredded cheese—serve with vegetables or croquettes. For creamed dishes, add ½–¾ cup cooked meat or flaked fish.

9

QUICK BREADS AND
YEAST BREADS

Quick Spelt Drop Biscuits

(No Egg, Milk)

---

2 cups spelt flour
1½ tablespoons baking powder
½ teaspoon salt
¼ cup vegetable oil
¾ cup water

Preheat oven to 425°F. Combine all ingredients in mixing bowl. Beat well. Drop by spoonfuls onto a lightly greased baking pan. Bake 10–12 minutes, or until browned on bottom.

Makes 12 servings.

One biscuit = 72   calories
               2 g   protein
              17 g   carbohydrates
               4 g   fat
             217 mg sodium

Pumpkin Bread

(No Wheat, Milk, Gluten)

2 cups brown rice flour
2 tablespoons potato or tapioca starch
½ teaspoon salt
2 teaspoons baking powder
¼ teaspoon baking soda
½ teaspoon ground cinnamon
¼ teaspoon ground nutmeg
¼ cup sugar
2 eggs
½ cup canned pumpkin
¼ cup vegetable oil
⅓ cup apple juice

Preheat oven to 350°F. Combine all ingredients in mixing bowl. Beat well until the batter is smooth and fluffy. Pour into an oiled 9" × 5" loaf pan. Bake 40–45 minutes. Cool in pan 10 minutes. Turn the pan over and set it on a wire rack. Let stand 5 minutes. Gently remove bread from the pan. Allow bread to cool thoroughly.

Makes 12 servings
One serving of 1 slice = 162   calories
3 g   protein
24 g   carbohydrates
6 g   fat
258 mg   sodium

❧

Eggless Pumpkin Date Bread

(No Wheat, Milk, Egg, Gluten)

½ *cup vegetable oil*
1 *cup firmly packed brown sugar*
1 *cup canned pumpkin*
1 *teaspoon vanilla extract*
1 *cup rice flour*
¼ *cup potato starch*
2 *teaspoons baking powder*
2 *teaspoons ground cinnamon*
½ *cup chopped dates*
½ *cup chopped nuts (if tolerated)*

Preheat oven to 350°F. Grease a 9″ × 5″ loaf pan. Combine oil, sugar, pumpkin, and vanilla in mixing bowl. Beat well. Sift dry ingredients and add them to the bowl. Mix just until all dry ingredients are moistened. Fold in dates and nuts. Pour batter into loaf pan and bake for 1 hour. Bread may be glazed with 1 cup sifted confectioners' sugar mixed with 2 tablespoons hot water if desired.

Makes 12 servings
One serving of 1 slice = 261   calories
3 g   protein
38 g   carbohydrates
14 g   fat
118 mg   sodium

Teff Pumpkin Bread

(No Wheat, Milk, Egg)

2 cups teff flour
¼ cup tapioca flour
2 teaspoons ground cinnamon
¼ teaspoon ground nutmeg
2 tablespoons baking powder
½ cup sugar
⅓ cup vegetable oil
1 cup canned pumpkin
1¼ cups apple juice
½ cup chopped nuts or dates

Preheat oven to 350°F. Combine all ingredients in mixing bowl. Mix thoroughly. Pour batter into 9″ × 13″ lightly oiled loaf pan. Bake 50–60 minutes, or until toothpick inserted into center comes out clean.

Makes 12 servings
One serving of 1 slice = 248   calories
4 g   protein
29 g   carbohydrates
8 g   fat
197 mg   sodium

❧

Garbanzo Skillet Bread

(No Wheat, Egg, Milk, Gluten)

⅓ cup water
¼ cup chickpea flour
¼ teaspoon salt
1 teaspoon olive oil

In a medium bowl mix water, flour, and salt with a whisk or fork. Set a 10-inch skillet on medium-high heat. When a drop of water dances on the skillet surface, add half the oil. Add batter all at once. Cover and cook for 2 minutes. Remove cover and dribble remaining oil over bread. Cook about 5 minutes more.

When the bread looks dry around the edges, use a spatula to flip it. Reduce heat to low and cook another 5 minutes uncovered. Remove to a wire rack. Let bread stand until you are ready to serve. Tear into irregular shapes.

Makes 1 serving

For additional servings, repeat single-batch recipe. Do not double recipe.

One serving = 96 calories
2 g protein
16 g carbohydrates
6 g fat
268 mg sodium

Orange Quinoa Muffins

(No Wheat, Egg, Milk)

1 pound quinoa flour (3⅔ cups)
1 teaspoon baking soda
½ teaspoon salt
Grated rind of 2 medium oranges
Juice of 2 medium oranges
¼ cup vegetable oil
½ cup maple syrup
¾ cup water

Preheat oven to 375°F. Stir flour, soda, and salt together. Add orange rind and juice. Stir in oil, syrup, and water. Mix until ingredients are blended. Spoon batter into muffin cups. Bake 18–22 minutes.

Makes 9 muffins
One muffin = 171   calories
                    2 g   protein
                  27 g   carbohydrates
                    7 g   fat
               208 mg   sodium

Oatmeal Scones

(No Wheat)

---

2 cups oat flour or ground oatmeal
2½ teaspoons baking powder
½ teaspoon baking soda
½ teaspoon salt
2 tablespoon sugar
½ cup butter or margarine
¾ cup buttermilk
1 egg

Preheat oven to 400°F. Sift together dry ingredients. Cut in butter until mixture resembles coarse cornmeal. Beat together buttermilk and egg, then add to dry ingredients, stirring with a fork until a stiff dough is formed. Knead lightly on board dusted with oat flour. Flatten into a round 1 inch thick and 5 inches in diameter; smooth out edges. Mark into 12 wedges with a knife. Place on ungreased baking sheet. Bake 10–12 minutes until lightly browned. Serve hot with butter and jelly.

Makes 12 servings
Once scone = 209 calories
4 g protein
31 g carbohydrates
11 g fat
291 mg sodium

Orange Barley Flour Bread

(No Wheat, Milk)

2 cups barley flour
½ cup sugar
½ teaspoon salt
3 teaspoons baking powder
2 eggs, beaten
½ cup orange juice
½ cup orange marmalade
¼ cup vegetable oil

Preheat oven to 350°F. Stir together dry ingredients. Add the rest of the ingredients. Beat well. Pour battter into lightly oiled 9″ × 5″ loaf pan. Bake 50–55 minutes. Cool 5 minutes in pan. Remove from pan and slice.

Makes 12 servings
One serving of 1 slice = 178   calories
3 g   protein
27 g   carbohydrates
7 g   fat
206 mg   sodium

✍

Rice-and-Barley Muffins

(No Wheat, Egg)

⅓ cup rice flour
⅔ cup barley flour
3 teaspoons baking powder
2 tablespoons sugar
¼ teaspoon salt
¾ cup milk
1 tablespoon vegetable oil

Preheat oven to 375°F. Mix dry ingredients together in bowl. Add milk and vegetable oil. Stir only enough to combine. Fill muffin pans two-thirds full. Bake 20 minutes, until lightly browned.

Makes 6 servings
One muffin = 155 calories
3 g protein
28 g carbohydrates
4 g fat
176 mg sodium

❧

Oat Biscuits

(No Wheat, Milk, Egg)

---

1 cup oat flour or ground oatmeal
½ teaspoon salt
3 teaspoons baking powder
1 tablespoon sugar
2 tablespoons shortening or milk-free
       margarine
⅓ cup cold water

Preheat oven to 400°F. Stir together dry ingredients; cut in shortening until size of peas. Add cold water; stir gently to form soft dough. Knead lightly on board dusted with oat flour. Roll out the dough to ½" thickness. Cut with 1½" cutter and place on ungreased baking sheet. Bake 15–20 minutes.

Makes 12 servings
One biscuit = 189   calories
              2 g   protein
             23 g   carbohydrates
             11 g   fat
            216 mg sodium

Chickpea Onion Bread

(No Wheat, Egg, Milk)

½ *cup finely chopped onion*
⅓ *cup olive oil*
1¾ *cups chickpea flour*
¼ *cup tapioca or arrowroot starch*
½ *teaspoon salt*
1 *tablespoon baking powder*
¾ *cup lukewarm water*

Preheat oven to 425°F. Sauté onion in the oil. Cook over medium-high heat, stirring, until the onion is soft but not brown. In a separate bowl, beat together the flour, starch, salt, and baking powder. Pour in water and the oil and onions. Mix well until the flour is moistened. Scrape batter into oiled 8-inch square pan and bake 18–20 minutes. When done, bread has a few cracks in the surface and the center feels crusty and firm. Let stand for 10–15 minutes before cutting.

Makes 8 servings
One serving of 1 slice = 167 calories
3 g protein
23 g carbohydrates
8 g fat
207 mg sodium

Teff Banana Muffins

(No Wheat, Milk)

2½ cups teff flour
1½ tablespoons baking powder
½ cup date sugar
1 teaspoon ground cinnamon
1½ cups water
¼ cup vegetable oil
2 bananas
1 egg

Preheat oven to 400°F. Combine flour, baking powder, sugar, and cinnamon in mixing bowl. Puree water, oil, bananas, and egg in a food processor. Add to the dry ingredients. Mix well. Spoon batter into muffin cups. Bake 10–15 minutes, or until done.

Makes 12 servings
One muffin = 175   calories
          3 g   protein
         30 g   carbohydrates
          7 g   fat
        129 mg sodium

Amaranth Muffins

(No Wheat, Egg, Milk)

---

2 cups amaranth flour
¼ cup arrowroot starch
1 tablespoon baking powder
¼ cup sugar
⅓ cup vegetable oil
¾ cup water

Preheat oven to 350°F. Combine flour, arrowroot, baking powder, and sugar in a bowl. Add oil and water. Stir until all ingredients are blended. Spoon batter into muffin cups and bake until tops are brown, about 25 minutes.

Makes 8 servings
One muffin = 169 calories
3 g protein
26 g carbohydrates
8 g fat
164 mg sodium

Banana Cinnamon Muffins

(No Wheat, Milk, Gluten)

¾ cup rice flour
¼ cup sweet rice flour
¼ cup rice polish
1 tablespoon baking powder
¼ teaspoon ground cinnamon
⅛ teaspoon ground nutmeg
1 tablespoon sugar
1 egg
½ banana, chopped fine
½ cup fruit juice
2 tablespoons vegetable oil

Preheat oven to 375°F. Combine flours, rice polish, baking powder, cinnamon, nutmeg, and sugar in a mixing bowl. Add the remaining ingredients and mix until well blended. Spoon into muffin cups. Bake 12–15 minutes or until muffin tops are browned.

Strawberry Muffins One cup sliced strawberries can be substituted for banana.

Makes 8 servings
One muffin = 97   calories
3 g   protein
19 g   carbohydrates
3 g   fat
191 mg   sodium

◈

Orange Oatmeal Bread

(No Wheat, Egg, Milk)

2¼ cups oat flour or ground oatmeal
4 teaspoons baking powder
¼ teaspoon baking soda
¾ cup sugar
¾ teaspoon salt
2 tablespoons vegetable oil
¾ cup orange juice
1 tablespoon grated orange rind

Preheat oven to 350°F. Sift together dry ingredients. Add oil, orange juice, and orange rind; stir until dry ingredients are moistened. Pour into a lightly oiled 9″ × 5″ loaf pan. Bake about 1 hour.

Makes 12 servings
One serving of 1 slice = 201   calories
                          3 g   protein
                         29 g   carbohydrates
                          8 g   fat
                       293 mg   sodium

Rye Bread

(No Wheat, Milk, Egg)

6 cups rye flour
1 tablespoon salt
2 packages dry yeast
½ cup instant mashed potatoes
2 cups hot water
½ cup molasses or honey
¼ cup vegetable oil

Preheat oven to 350°F. In large mixing bowl thoroughly blend 2 cups flour, salt, and yeast. In a separate bowl, combine instant mashed potatoes and hot water. Whip lightly with a fork. Combine molasses, oil, potato, and water. Add this mixture to the dry ingredients. Beat 2 minutes at medium speed, scraping bowl occasionally. Add 2 cups flour. Beat at high speed 2 minutes, scraping the sides of the bowl occasionally. Stir in the remaining 2 cups flour (or enough to make a stiff dough). Sprinkle bread board with rye flour. Turn dough out and knead until smooth and elastic (8–10 minutes). Place dough in greased bowl; cover and let rise in a warm place until it is doubled in bulk (1½–2 hours). Grease two 9″ × 5″ loaf pans. Punch down dough and shape into two loaves. Cover and let rise until it is doubled in bulk (30–45 minutes). Bake 40 minutes, or until loaves sound hollow when tapped lightly.

Makes 2 large loaves
One serving of 1 slice = 111 calories
2 g protein
16 g carbohydrates
4 g fat
317 mg sodium

❧

Rice Bran Muffins

(No Wheat, Gluten)

---

1 cup brown rice flour
½ cup rice bran
2 tablespoons sugar
1 tablespoon baking powder
½ teaspoon salt
¼ cup vegetable oil
2 eggs
¾ cup milk or apple juice

Preheat oven to 400°F. Combine all ingredients in a bowl. Beat well until batter is smooth. Pour into lightly oiled muffin cups. Bake 12–15 minutes.

Makes 6 servings
One muffin = 118 calories
3 g protein
21 g carbohydrates
6 g fat
247 mg sodium

Blueberry Muffins

(No Wheat, Milk, Gluten)

1 cup brown rice flour
½ cup rice bran
1½ teaspoons baking powder
1 egg
2 tablespoons vegetable oil
1 tablespoon honey
¾ cup orange juice or water
½ cup blueberries

Preheat oven to 400°F. Combine flour, bran, and baking powder in bowl. Stir to mix. Add rest of the ingredients. Mix well. Spoon into lightly greased muffin cups. Bake 12–15 minutes or until brown.

Prune Plum Muffins ½ cup chopped Italian prune plums can be substituted for blueberries.

Makes 9 servings
One muffin = 151   calories
3 g   protein
21 g   carbohydrates
8 g   fat
194 mg   sodium

❧

Rice Flour Strawberry Muffins

(No Wheat, Milk, Gluten)

¾ *cup brown rice flour*
¼ *cup sweet rice flour*
¼ *cup rice polish*
1 *tablespoon baking powder*
¼ *teaspoon ground nutmeg*
1 *tablespoon honey*
2 *tablespoons vegetable oil*
1 *egg*
1 *cup sliced fresh strawberries*
½ *cup orange juice or water*

Preheat oven to 350°F. Combine rice flours, rice polish, baking powder, and nutmeg in mixing bowl. Stir to blend. Add the remaining ingredients and mix until well blended. Spoon into lightly oiled muffin cups. Bake 15–18 minutes, or until brown.

Makes 8 servings
One muffin = 148 calories
2 g protein
22 g carbohydrates
6 g fat
203 mg sodium

Rice Banana Spice Muffins

(No Wheat, Egg, Milk, Gluten)

1 very ripe banana, cut into 1/4-inch pieces
1/4 cup vegetable oil
1/3 cup rice beverage or water
1/2 cup sugar
2 cups brown rice flour
3 tablespoons arrowroot powder
1 tablespoon baking powder
1 teaspoon ground cinnamon
1/2 teaspoon ground nutmeg

Preheat oven to 400°F. Cream together banana, oil, and rice beverage. Add sugar. Stir in remaining ingredients. Beat well. Spoon into lightly greased muffin cups. Bake 15–18 minutes.

Makes 9 servings
One muffin = 156   calories
2 g   protein
24 g   carbohydrates
6 g   fat
204 mg   sodium

Rice Flour Muffins with Egg

(No Wheat, Milk, Gluten)

---

1 cup rice flour
3 tablespoons soy flour
¼ teaspoon salt
2 tablespoons sugar
2 teaspoons baking powder
¾ cup orange or apple juice
1 egg
2 tablespoons vegetable oil

Preheat oven to 375°F. Combine rice flour, soy flour, salt, sugar, and baking powder into mixing bowl. Stir to blend. Add orange juice, egg, and oil. Mix until smooth. Pour into lightly oiled muffin tins. Bake 15 minutes.

Date Muffins Add ½ cup dates to batter just before pouring into muffin tins.

Blueberry Muffins Add ½ cup fresh or frozen blueberries to batter just before pouring into muffin tins.

Makes 8 servings
One muffin = 136   calories
3 g   protein
18 g   carbohydrates
7 g   fat
201 mg   sodium

ॐ

Rice Flour Muffins Without Egg

(No Wheat, Egg, Milk, Gluten)

⅓ cup rice polish
¼ cup rice flour
1 tablespoon potato starch
½ teaspoon arrowroot
¼ teaspoon salt
2 teaspoons baking powder
1 tablespoon honey
⅓ cup orange juice
¼ cup water
2 tablespoons vegetable oil

Preheat oven to 375°F. Combine rice polish, rice flour, potato starch, arrowroot, salt, and baking powder in mixing bowl. Stir to blend ingredients. Add honey, orange juice, water, and oil. Beat until all ingredients are combined. Pour batter into lightly oiled muffin cups. Bake 12–15 minutes.

Makes 6 servings
One muffin = 128   calories
             2 g   protein
            17 g   carbohydrates
             6 g   fat
           291 mg sodium

Oatmeal Shortbread

(No Wheat, Egg, Milk)

½ cup margarine
½ cup sugar
1¼ cups oat flour or ground oatmeal

Preheat oven to 350°F. Cream margarine and sugar until light. Add oat flour gradually to make a crumbly mixture. Press together and shape into a smooth ball. Divide dough into four parts. On lightly floured (oat flour) board, roll each part into a 6-inch circle. Place them 4″ apart on lightly oiled baking sheets. Mark each circle into eight wedges. Bake 15 minutes.

Makes 30 servings
One cookie =   162   calories
              2 g   protein
              21 g   carbohydrates
              8 g   fat
              61 mg   sodium

Corn Muffins or Cornbread with Egg

(No Wheat, Milk, Gluten)

2 cups cornmeal
¼ teaspoon salt
3 teaspoons baking powder
1 tablespoon sugar
2 eggs
2 tablespoons vegetable oil
¾ cup water

Preheat oven to 400°F. Combine all ingredients in mixing bowl. Beat thoroughly to blend. Pour into lightly oiled muffin tins or 8-inch square baking pan. Bake 15–20 minutes or until golden brown.

Makes 9 servings
One muffin = 118   calories
            3 g   protein
           20 g   carbohydrates
            3 g   fat
          218 mg sodium

❧

Cornbread Without Egg

(No Wheat, Egg, Milk)

---

2 cups cornmeal
¼ cup tapioca flour
¼ cup maple syrup or honey
¾ cup rice beverage or water
¼ cup vegetable oil
1 tablespoon baking powder

Preheat oven to 375°F. Combine all ingredients in mixing bowl. Beat just until blended. Pour into lightly oiled 8-inch square pan. Bake 15–20 minutes, or until golden brown on top and sides pull away from pan.

Makes 8 servings
One serving = 168   calories
              2 g   protein
             25 g   carbohydrates
              7 g   fat
           182 mg   sodium

Quick Rice Bran Bread

(No Wheat, Gluten)

2 eggs
2 tablespoons vegetable oil
2 tablespoons sugar
¾ cup milk
1⅓ cups brown rice flour
¼ cup soy flour
½ cup rice bran
½ teaspoon salt
2 teaspoons baking powder
½ teaspoon baking soda

Preheat oven to 350°F. Cream together eggs, oil, and sugar. Slowly add milk alternately with rest of the ingredients. Beat well. (This mixture cannot be overbeaten.) Pour batter into lightly oiled 9″ × 5″ loaf pan. Bake 40–45 minutes or until browned.

Raisin Bread Add ⅓ cup chopped raisins or currants.

Orange Date Bread Add 1 tablespoon grated orange rind and ⅓ cup chopped dates.

Banana Bread Add 2 very ripe, pureed bananas and reduce milk to ½ cup.

Makes 12 servings
One serving of 1 slice = 142   calories
3 g   protein
18 g   carbohydrates
7 g   fat
314 mg   sodium

Ozark Corn Pone

(No Wheat, Milk, Egg, Gluten)

---

1 cup cornmeal
½ teaspoon salt
1 cup boiling water
2 teaspoons melted shortening or
*   vegetable oil*

Preheat oven to 450°F. Combine cornmeal, salt, and boiling water. Stir to form a stiff dough. Rinse hands in cold water. Shape dough into two flat, ½-inch thick, oval cakes. Place on lightly oiled baking sheet. Brush with oil or melted shortening. Bake 20 minutes or until brown and crisp. Cut into 12 pieces and serve as bread substitute.

Makes 12 servings
One serving = 82 calories
               2 g protein
              14 g carbohydrates
               2 g fat
              26 mg sodium

Spicy Cornbread

(No Wheat, Gluten)

¾ cup rice flour
1 cup cornmeal
2 tablespoons sugar
2 teaspoons baking powder
½ teaspoon baking soda
½ teaspoon salt
½ teaspoon chili powder
¼ teaspoon ground cumin
¼ cup pimento
1 cup yogurt
1 egg
3 tablespoons oil
3 tablespoons finely chopped scallions

Preheat oven to 400°F. Stir together the rice flour, cornmeal, sugar, baking powder, baking soda, salt, chili powder, and cumin. Cut the pimento into ¼-inch pieces and stir into dry ingredients. Using a separate bowl, combine the yogurt with remaining ingredients and stir into dry ingredients until just blended. Pour into a buttered 8-inch skillet. Bake approximately 20–25 minutes, until toothpick inserted into center comes out clean. Serve warm or cooled.

Makes 8 servings
One serving = 139   calories
              3 g   protein
              18 g   carbohydrates
              6 g   fat
              289 mg sodium

Banana Cornmeal Spoonbread

(No Wheat, Gluten)

---

2 medium ripe bananas, peeled
4 eggs, separated
1 cup milk
3 tablespoons butter
1 cup cornmeal
1 teaspoon baking powder
¾ teaspoon salt
¼ teaspoon cream of tartar

Preheat oven to 350°F. Slice bananas into blender container; process until pureed. Beat egg yolks until thick and lemon-colored, 3–5 minutes. Combine bananas, milk, and butter in large saucepan. Cook on medium heat until butter melts. Stir in cornmeal, baking powder, and salt. Cook, stirring constantly, until mixture thickens, about 3 minutes. Remove from heat. Beat in egg yolks. In a separate bowl combine egg whites and cream of tartar and beat until stiff but not dry. Fold into the banana mixture. Pour into well oiled 1½ quart casserole. Bake 30–35 minutes or until knife inserted in the middle comes out clean.

Makes 4 servings
One serving = 216 calories
                3 g protein
            28 g carbohydrates
            12 g fat
        357 mg sodium

❧

Potato Biscuits

(No Wheat, Egg, Gluten)

½ cup potato starch flour
3 teaspoons baking powder
¼ teaspoon salt
3 tablespoons shortening or butter
¼ cup milk

Preheat oven to 425°F. Stir together dry ingredients. Cut in shortening until size of peas. Slowly add milk, stirring gently to form soft dough. Lightly dust a bread board with potato flour. Turn the dough out onto the board and knead lightly. Roll to ½-inch thickness. Using a ½-inch cutter, cut out nine biscuits and place on an ungreased baking sheet. Bake 10–12 minutes, until lightly browned.

Makes 9 servings
One biscuit = 86   calories
              2 g   protein
             11 g   carbohydrates
              4 g   fat
            211 mg   sodium

Rice Flour Yeast Bread

(No Wheat, Gluten)

3 cups rice flour
½ cup potato starch flour
2 packages dry yeast
2 tablespoons sugar
1 teaspoon salt
2 tablespoons baking powder
1 cup dry milk
¼ cup instant mashed potatoes
2 cups very hot water
¼ cup soft butter or margarine
4 eggs, beaten

Stir flours together. Measure 2 cups into large mixer bowl. Add dry yeast, sugar, salt, baking powder, and dry milk. Mix thoroughly. Combine instant mashed potatoes and hot water; whip lightly with a fork. Add potato mixture and soft butter to dry ingredients in mixer bowl. Beat 3 minutes on medium speed. Add remaining flour and eggs; beat 3 minutes on medium speed. Mixture will resemble thick cake batter. Leave batter in bowl; cover and let rise in warm place for 1 hour. Batter will rise about 2 inches depending on size of bowl. Beat just enough to remove large gas bubbles. Preheat oven to 325°F. Lightly oil two 9″ × 5″ loaf pans. Pour batter into pans; cover and let rise 30 minutes. Bake 30–35 minutes, until lightly browned.

Makes 24 servings
One serving of 1 slice = 120   calories
3 g   protein
18 g   carbohydrates
4 g   fat
314 mg   sodium

❧

Rice Crackers

(No Wheat, Egg, Milk, Gluten)

1 cup rice flour
½ teaspoon salt
½ cup potato starch
½ cup margarine
½ cup cold water

Preheat oven to 400°F. Combine rice flour, salt, and potato starch in mixing bowl. Cut in margarine with pastry blender or fork. Stir in enough cold water to make soft dough. Place dough on lightly oiled baking sheet. Cover with waxed paper and roll with rolling pin to ⅛-inch thickness. Cut into 48 squares. Bake 10–15 minutes.

Sesame Rice Crackers Add 1 tablespoon toasted sesame seeds to dough before rolling out onto baking sheet.

Poppy Seed Rice Crackers Add 1 tablespoon toasted poppy seeds to dough before rolling out onto baking sheet.

Parmesan Rice Crackers Add 1 tablespoon grated Parmesan cheese to dough before rolling out onto baking sheet.

Makes 12 servings
One serving of 4 crackers = 137   calories
                            2 g   protein
                           12 g   carbohydrates
                            9 g   fat
                          216 mg sodium

High-Fiber Rice Waffles or Pancakes

(No Wheat, Gluten)

1 cup brown rice flour
1/2 cup rice bran
1/4 cup soy flour
2 teaspoons baking powder
2 teaspoons sugar
1/2 teaspoon salt
2 eggs
3 tablespoons vegetable oil
3/4 cup milk

Combine all ingredients in mixing bowl. Beat until smooth. Pour into lightly oiled waffle iron or oiled griddle. Remove from waffle iron or turn pancakes when browned.

Makes 4 waffles or 8 pancakes
One serving
(1 waffle or 2 large pancakes) = 141   calories
                              3 g   protein
                             16 g   carbohydrates
                              8 g   fat
                            297 mg   sodium

Cornmeal Pancakes or Waffles

(No Wheat, Milk, Gluten)

---

1 cup cornmeal
1/4 cup soy or tapioca flour
1/4 teaspoon salt
2 tablespoons sugar
1 1/2 teaspoons baking powder
3/4 cup water
1 teaspoon vegetable oil
1 egg

Combine all ingredients in bowl. Beat until smooth. Pour batter onto lightly oiled griddle or waffle iron. Remove from waffle iron or turn pancakes when browned.

Makes 6 pancakes or 2 waffles
One serving (1 waffle or 3 pancakes) = 96 calories
                                      4 g protein
                                     16 g carbohydrates
                                      2 g fat
                                    187 mg sodium

Buckwheat Pancakes

(No Wheat, Milk, Egg)

---

1 package dry yeast
1 tablespoon brown sugar
2 cups buckwheat flour
½ cup cornmeal
1 teaspoon salt
2½ cups hot water
1 teaspoon baking soda
1 teaspoon warm water
2 tablespoons vegetable oil

In mixer bowl, thoroughly combine all dry ingredients except baking soda. Add hot water. Beat 2 minutes on medium speed. Cover and allow to rise overnight in warm place. In the morning, stir the mixture well. Add baking soda dissolved in warm water and oil; mix again. Cook on hot greased griddle until dry around edges. Turn. Remove from heat when browned. Serve with syrup.

Makes 5 servings
One serving of 3 pancakes = 142   calories
2 g   protein
16 g   carbohydrates
8 g   fat
267 mg   sodium

10

CAKES AND DESSERTS

Rice Flour Applesauce Cake

(No Wheat, Milk, Egg)

---

2 cups brown rice flour
1/4 cup arrowroot flour
1/2 cup sugar
1 tablespoon baking powder
1 teaspoon ground cinnamon
1/2 teaspoon ground nutmeg
1/2 cup applesauce
1/2 cup apple juice
1/3 cup vegetable oil

Preheat oven to 375°F. Combine all ingredients in mixing bowl. Pour batter into lightly oiled 8-inch square baking pan. Bake 15–20 minutes. Cool. Cut into squares.

Makes 12 servings
One serving =   164   calories
                2 g   protein
               27 g   carbohydrates
                6 g   fat
              185 mg sodium

Spelt Flour Plum Coffeecake

(No Wheat, Egg, Milk)

12–15 small prune plums
⅓ cup date sugar
2 tablespoons spelt flour
2¾ cups spelt flour, ground fine
1 tablespoon baking powder
½ teaspoon salt
½ cup honey
½ cup water or Nut Milk (See Index.)
¼ cup oil

Preheat oven to 350°F. Quarter and pit plums, using enough to cover bottom of an oiled 8-inch square baking dish in a single layer. Sprinkle with date sugar and 2 tablespoons of spelt flour. Toss fruit lightly to coat. Spread mixture evenly on bottom of pan. Place 2¾ cups flour into a mixing bowl. Add baking powder and salt. Stir to blend. Pour honey, water, and oil into a 2-cup glass container. Stir to combine. Pour liquids over the flour mixture. Beat until all flour is moistened. Pour batter over plum mixture, spreading it evenly into corners. Bake 30–35 minutes, until top is brown and firm. This recipe can be served hot or cold. To serve, slice and then lift with a spatula and flip each portion over onto a plate, turning the gooey fruit side up.

Makes 8 servings
One serving = 176   calories
                2 g   protein
               31 g   carbohydrates
                6 g   fat
              307 mg sodium

~~

Teff Applesauce Cake

(No Wheat, Milk, Gluten)

---

1 cup teff flour
1 cup rice flour
¼ cup arrowroot
1 teaspoon ground cinnamon
¼ teaspoon ground nutmeg
1 tablespoon baking powder
1 cup applesauce
½ cup vegetable oil
½ cup honey
2 eggs

Preheat oven to 350°F. Combine teff flour, rice flour, arrowroot, cinnamon, nutmeg, and baking powder in mixing bowl. Stir to blend. Add applesauce, oil, honey, and eggs. Mix well. Pour into oiled 8-inch square baking pan. Bake 30–35 minutes, or until toothpick inserted into center comes out clean.

Makes 16 servings
One serving = 179   calories
   3 g   protein
   29 g   carbohydrates
   7 g   fat
   199 mg   sodium

Amaranth Cake

(No Wheat, Egg, Milk)

---

2 cups amaranth flour
1 tablespoon baking powder
¼ cup arrowroot
½ cup sugar
½ cup vegetable oil
1 cup water or apple juice
½ teaspoon allspice
⅓ cup finely chopped walnuts

Preheat oven to 375°F. Stir together all ingredients in a medium bowl. Beat well. Pour batter into oiled 8-inch square pan. Bake 25–30 minutes. Cool thoroughly. Dust with confectioners' sugar just before serving.

Makes 9 servings
One serving = 181 calories
            2 g protein
            25 g carbohydrates
            8 g fat
            205 mg sodium

◦✒

Rhubarb Crumble

(No Wheat, Egg, Milk, Gluten)

———————

2 cups chopped rhubarb
¼ cup water
2 tablespoons cream of rice cereal, uncooked
¼ cup brown sugar
2 tablespoons soy milk powder
2 tablespoons vegetable oil
¼ teaspoon cinnamon

Preheat oven to 350°F. Put rhubarb in casserole dish and add water. Sprinkle on cream of rice cereal. In a separate bowl combine brown sugar, soy milk powder, vegetable oil, and cinnamon to make streusel topping. Drop topping over rhubarb mixture. Bake about 30 minutes or until fruit is tender. Serve hot or cold.

Makes 3 servings
One serving = 234 calories
            2 g protein
           34 g carbohydrates
           11 g fat
           87 mg sodium

❧

Banana Snack Cake

(No Wheat, Milk, Gluten)

---

2 ripe bananas
½ cup sugar
3 eggs
½ cup vegetable oil
2 cups brown rice flour
1 tablespoon baking powder

Preheat oven to 375°F. Puree bananas, sugar, eggs, and oil in food processor or blender. Stir in flour and baking powder. Pour into oiled 9-inch square baking pan. Bake 30–35 minutes.

Makes 8 servings
One serving = 241 calories
              3 g protein
             31 g carbohydrates
             12 g fat
            251 mg sodium

❧

Pineapple Upside-Down Cake

(No Wheat, Egg, Gluten)

---

1 tablespoon plus ⅓ cup margarine
½ cup brown sugar
1 8-ounce can crushed pineapple
(juice packed)
⅓ cup sugar
⅔ cup pineapple juice
1 cup rice flour
1 tablespoon potato or tapioca starch
2 teaspoons baking powder
⅛ teaspoon salt
1 teaspoon vanilla extract

Preheat oven to 350°F. In a small saucepan, melt 1 tablespoon margarine and brown sugar. Pour into 9-inch square cake pan. Drain pineapple juice into a small bowl. Arrange the crushed pineapple on top of the sugar mixture. Prepare cake batter by creaming together ⅓ cup sugar and ⅓ cup margarine. Add pineapple juice, rice flour, starch, baking powder, salt, and vanilla extract. Beat well. Pour batter over pineapple mixture. Bake 20–30 minutes, or until cake is done.

Makes 6 servings
One serving = 248   calories
              2 g   protein
             32 g   carbohydrates
             13 g   fat
            310 mg sodium

Pear Cobbler

(No Wheat, Egg, Milk, Gluten)

COBBLER BASE

> *4 medium-size pears, sliced*
> *¼ teaspoon cinnamon*
> *Dash of cloves*
> *Dash of nutmeg*
> *2 tablespoons frozen orange juice*
>   *concentrate, melted*

TOPPING

> *½ cup brown rice flour*
> *1½ teaspoons baking powder*
> *3 tablespoons margarine*
> *2–3 tablespoons cold water*

Preheat oven to 400°F. Line a lightly oiled casserole dish with sliced pears. Sprinkle on spices and drizzle orange juice concentrate over pear slices. Bake 5 minutes while preparing topping.

Combine flour and baking powder in mixing bowl. Cut in margarine to resemble pie crust mixture. Add water and stir with fork. Crumble mixture on top of pear slices. Bake 15 minutes longer. Cool and serve.

Makes 4 servings
One serving = 202　calories
　　　　　　　2 g　protein
　　　　　　24 g　carbohydrates
　　　　　　12 g　fat
　　　　290 mg　sodium

Apple Crisp

(No Wheat, Egg, Milk, Gluten)

---

4 medium apples, thinly sliced (about 3 cups)
¼ cup apple juice
1 tablespoon honey
2 tablespoons soy flour
¼ cup rice flour
½ teaspoon cinnamon
2 tablespoons vegetable oil

Preheat oven to 350°F. Place apple slices in lightly oiled 8-inch square baking pan. Pour on apple juice. Drizzle honey over apples. Combine soy and rice flours in mixing bowl with cinnamon. Add vegetable oil and toss lightly. The mixture should be dry and crumbly. Sprinkle mixture over apples. Bake 20 minutes or until top is lightly browned.

Makes 4 servings
One serving = 148 calories
2 g protein
22 g carbohydrates
7 g fat
184 mg sodium

Almond Oatmeal Torte

(No Wheat, Milk)

6 eggs, separated
1 cup sugar
1 teaspoon orange extract
1 teaspoon almond extract
1 cup finely ground almonds*
⅓ cup ground oatmeal
¼ teaspoon salt
½ cup prepared lemon pie filling
Confectioners' sugar

Preheat oven to 350°F. Beat egg yolks and ½ cup sugar together until thick and lemon-colored. Stir in extracts, ground almonds, and oatmeal. Beat egg whites and salt in a separate bowl until soft peaks form. Gradually add the remaining ½ cup sugar and beat until stiff peaks form. Fold the egg yolk mixture into the egg whites. Divide batter into three 9-inch layer cake pans lined with waxed paper. Bake 30 minutes. Cool before removing from pans. Put layers together with lemon pie filling. Dust with confectioners' sugar or top with nondairy dessert topping.

Makes 12 servings
One serving = 157   calories
            5 g   protein
           21 g   carbohydrates
            7 g   fat
          312 mg   sodium

You can buy ground almonds or whole. If you buy whole almonds, grind them in a blender or food processor.

❧

Chocolate Cake

(No Wheat, Gluten)

½ cup margarine
⅔ cup sugar
2 eggs
1 teaspoon vanilla
6 tablespoons cocoa
2 cups rice flour
1 teaspoon baking powder
½ teaspoon baking soda
½ cup yogurt

Preheat oven to 350°F. Cream margarine and sugar. Beat in eggs until the mixture is light and fluffy. Add vanilla and cocoa. Beat in rice flour sifted together with baking powder and baking soda just until blended. Blend in yogurt. Pour into 8-inch square cake pan. Bake approximately 20 minutes.

Makes 8 servings
One serving = 231 calories
2 g protein
31 g carbohydrates
12 g fat
236 mg sodium

Chocolate Cream Roll

(No Wheat, Milk, Gluten)

3 eggs, separated
⅓ cup sugar
¼ cup cocoa
2 teaspoons potato flour

Preheat oven to 350°F. Separate eggs. Beat yolks with sugar, cocoa, and potato flour. Using a separate bowl, beat egg whites until they are stiff. Fold into chocolate mixture. Line the bottom of 13″ × 9″ pan with waxed paper. Pour batter into pan. Bake 10–15 minutes or until done. Cool in pan 5–10 minutes. Lay out a clean towel and sprinkle it with powdered sugar. Turn cake out onto the towel. Gently pull off waxed paper. Roll up jelly roll fashion, using the towel to wrap the cake. Let cool at least 2 hours. Unroll cake and spread with nondairy topping or frozen soy dessert. Reroll. Refrigerate or freeze until ready to serve. Keep wrapped to prevent drying out.

Makes 9 servings
One serving (without filling) = 108   calories
                                        3 g   protein
                                    18 g   carbohydrates
                                        3 g   fat
                                118 mg   sodium

✑

Chocolate Truffles

(No Wheat, Egg, Gluten)

⅓ cup heavy cream
6 ounces semisweet chocolate broken
   into small pieces
1 tablespoon softened unsalted butter
   or margarine
¼ cup unsweetened cocoa powder

Heat cream just to boiling in saucepan. Remove from heat and add chocolate and butter. Stir until chocolate is melted. Pour mixture into shallow pie plate or casserole dish. Cover with plastic wrap and refrigerate 3–4 hours. Dust a cutting board with a thin layer of cocoa. Scoop chocolate mixture into 24 small teaspoonfuls. Form each into a ball and roll it in cocoa. Place in waxed-paper-lined box or container. Cover and refrigerate until ready to serve.

Makes 24 truffles
One serving = 186   calories
          1 g   protein
         12 g   carbohydrates
         18 g   fat
        147 mg sodium

❧

Flourless Chocolate Cake

(No Wheat, Gluten)

CAKE

> 8 ounces unsalted margarine or butter
> ⅔ cup plus 1 tablespoon sugar
> 6 egg yolks
> 8 ounces high-quality semisweet chocolate,
>   melted
> 8 ounces almonds, ground
> 6 egg whites
> Pinch of cream of tartar

Preheat oven to 350°F. Line bottom of 9-inch, 3-inch deep spring-form pan with parchment or silicon paper.

Cream margarine with ⅓ cup plus 1 tablespoon sugar until light and fluffy. Add egg yolks to creamed mixture and beat well. Blend in chocolate, then ground almonds. Using a separate bowl whip egg whites with cream of tartar until frothy. Sprinkle in the remaining ⅓ cup of sugar, and continue to beat until soft peaks form. Gently fold egg whites into chocolate mixture until folded in evenly.

Pour cake mixture into pan. Bake 55–70 minutes. When toothpick inserted in center comes out clean, the cake is done. Let cool in the pan while you prepare the frosting.

FROSTING

> *12 ounces high-quality bittersweet chocolate,*
> *chopped fine*
> *1 cup of heavy cream*

Put chocolate in a large mixing bowl. Scald cream in a saucepan and pour through a sieve over chocolate. Let mixture stand for 1 minute to allow chocolate to soften. Beat until the frosting appears smooth and glossy.

   Invert cake onto plate. Peel parchment from bottom. Frost top and sides of cake and allow to set 1–2 hours.

Makes 12 servings
One serving = 348 calories
          3 g protein
      36 g carbohydrates
      18 g fat
   274 mg sodium

Fudge Soy Flour Cake

(No Wheat, Milk, Egg, Gluten)

1 cup soy flour
½ cup potato starch flour
½ cup sugar
¼ cup cocoa
½ teaspoon salt
2 teaspoons baking powder
1 teaspoon baking soda
1 teaspoon vanilla extract
1 tablespoon vinegar
½ cup vegetable oil
1 cup cold water

Preheat oven to 325°F. Stir together all dry ingredients in mixing bowl. Add remaining ingredients. Beat at medium speed for 3 minutes until batter is very smooth. Pour into lightly oiled 8-inch square baking pan. Bake 40 minutes. Cool cake in pan.

Makes 12 servings
One serving = 162 calories
            4 g protein
           24 g carbohydrates
            6 g fat
          349 mg sodium

❧

Orange Sponge Roll

(No Wheat, Milk, Gluten)

---

3 eggs
⅓ cup sugar
⅓ cup brown rice flour
2 teaspoons potato flour
1 tablespoon grated orange rind
2 teaspoons baking powder

Preheat oven to 350°F. Combine all ingredients in mixing bowl. Beat well. Line bottom of 13″ × 9″ pan with waxed paper. Pour batter into pan. Bake 10–15 minutes or until done. Cool in pan 5–10 minutes. Lay out a clean towel and sprinkle it with powdered sugar. Turn cake out onto the towel. Gently pull off waxed paper. Roll up jelly roll fashion, using the towel to wrap the cake. Let cool at least 2 hours. Unroll cake and spread with nondairy topping or frozen soy dessert. Reroll. Refrigerate or freeze until ready to serve. Keep wrapped to prevent drying out.

Makes 9 servings
One serving = 118 calories
 3 g protein
 19 g carbohydrates
 3 g fat
 127 mg sodium

Pecan Cups

(No Wheat, Gluten)

½ cup soft butter or margarine
3 ounces softened cream cheese
1¼ cups rice flour
½ teaspoon cinnamon
1 egg, well beaten
¾ cup brown sugar
1 cup chopped pecans
2 tablespoons melted butter or margarine
¼ teaspoon salt
½ teaspoon vanilla
¼ teaspoon nutmeg

Preheat oven to 350°F. Cream butter and cream cheese. Stir in flour and cinnamon until well blended. Divide into 12 walnut-sized balls. Press into greased muffin tins.

Combine egg, brown sugar, pecans, butter, salt, vanilla, and nutmeg in a mixing bowl. Spoon into muffin cups. Each should be about ¾ full. Bake 30 minutes.

Makes 12 servings
One serving = 297   calories
2 g   protein
37 g   carbohydrates
16 g   fat
297 mg   sodium

&

Cream Puffs

(No Wheat, Gluten)

¼ cup water
¼ cup butter or margarine
½ cup brown rice flour
2 teaspoons potato starch
2 eggs

Preheat oven to 400 °F. Combine water and butter in saucepan. Heat until butter is melted. Add flour and potato starch. Beat well. Add one egg at a time. Beat well until dough is shiny and smooth. Drop by tablespoonfuls onto oiled baking sheet, leaving about 2 inches between each. Bake 30–35 minutes, or until light and golden brown. Remove from oven. Cut off top to allow steam to escape. When cool, fill with whipped cream or vanilla custard. Top with chocolate frosting or powdered sugar before serving.

Makes 8 servings
One serving = 78 calories
2 g protein
14 g carbohydrates
8 g fat
188 mg sodium

Oatmeal Banana Cake

(No Wheat, Milk)

2 cups oat flour or ground oatmeal
3 teaspoons baking powder
1 teaspoon baking soda
1/4 teaspoon salt
1 cup sugar
3 eggs
1/2 cup vegetable oil
1 teaspoon vanilla extract
1 1/2 cups mashed banana
1/2 cup chopped dates
1/2 cup chopped nuts (if tolerated)

Preheat oven to 350°F. Stir together dry ingredients in a mixing bowl. Add eggs, oil, vanilla, and mashed banana. Beat until smooth. Stir in chopped dates and nuts. Pour into lightly oiled 8-inch square pan. Bake 25–30 minutes. Cool. Dust with confectioners' sugar.

Makes 9 servings
One serving = 237   calories
3 g   protein
38 g   carbohydrates
7 g   fat
208 mg   sodium

✤

Raisin Oatmeal Cake

(No Wheat, Milk)

1 cup hot water
1 cup oatmeal
½ cup raisins
¼ cup vegetable oil
½ cup molasses
2 eggs, beaten
1 cup oat flour or ground oatmeal
3 teaspoons baking powder
¼ teaspoon baking soda
½ cup chopped pecans or walnuts (optional)

Preheat oven to 350°F. Pour hot water over oatmeal and raisins. Stir. Add all remaining ingredients. Beat until thoroughly mixed. Pour into lightly oiled 9″ × 5″ loaf pan. Bake 45 minutes until lightly browned.

Makes 12 servings
One serving = 172 calories
3 g protein
27 g carbohydrates
6 g fat
202 mg sodium

Barley Banana Spice Cake

(No Wheat, Egg, Milk)

2¼ cups barley flour
1 cup sugar
1 tablespoon baking powder
1 teaspoon cinnamon
¼ teaspoon cloves
¼ teaspoon allspice
2 cups pureed or very well-mashed bananas
⅓ cup vegetable oil

Preheat oven to 375°F. In large bowl combine dry ingredients. In a small bowl, combine the bananas and oil. Stir liquids into dry ingredients until just mixed. Pour into oiled and floured 8-inch square pan. Bake 25–30 minutes, or until lightly brown and a toothpick inserted in center comes out dry.

Makes 8 servings
One serving = 182   calories
               2 g   protein
            29 g   carbohydrates
              7 g   fat
        218 mg   sodium

⊰⊱

Pumpkin Pie

(No Wheat, Egg, Milk, Gluten)

PIE

> 2 cups canned or cooked pumpkin
> ½ cup firmly packed brown sugar
> 1½ cups water or soy milk
> 6 tablespoons cornstarch or tapioca starch
> ½ teaspoon salt
> 1 teaspoon pumpkin pie spice
> 1 9-inch unbaked rice pie crust

Preheat oven to 375°F. Combine pumpkin, sugar, water or soy milk, cornstarch or tapioca, salt, and pumpkin pie spice in medium saucepan. Cook over low heat, stirring constantly, until mixture begins to thicken. Pour into pie crust. Bake 30 minutes.

CRUNCHY TOPPING

> ¼ cup brown sugar, packed firmly
> ¼ cup coconut, shredded
> ¼ cup chopped pecans (if tolerated)

Combine ingredients for crunchy topping and sprinkle on top of pie. Bake 5 minutes more.

Makes 7 servings
One serving = 279   calories
           3 g   protein
         36 g   carbohydrates
         14 g   fat
     382 mg   sodium

Pineapple Date Cake

(No Wheat, Milk, Egg, Gluten)

1 can (1 pound) crushed pineapple,
   undrained
1 cup firmly packed brown sugar
1/2 cup vegetable oil
3/4 cup water
1 1/2 cups raisins
1/2 cup chopped dates
3 tablespoons instant mashed-potato mix or
   2 tablespoons potato starch
1 tablespoon pumpkin pie spice
   (or spices tolerated)
1 1/4 cups rice flour
1/2 cup soy flour
1 teaspoon baking soda
2 teaspoons baking powder
1/2 cup chopped nuts (if tolerated)

Preheat oven to 325°F. In a 3-quart saucepan mix together the pineapple, brown sugar, oil, and water. Add raisins, dates, instant potato mix, and pumpkin pie spice. Mix well.

Place the mixture over medium heat and bring to a boil. Simmer, uncovered, for 5 minutes. Remove from heat and add rice flour. Stir well. Cool. Sift together soy flour, baking soda, and baking powder. Add to cooked mixture; mix thoroughly. Add nuts. Pour into lightly oiled 9″ × 13″ baking pan and bake 1 hour. When cool, dust with confectioners' sugar. This is a very moist cake.

Makes 15 servings
One serving = 214 calories
 3 g protein
 33 g carbohydrates
 8 g fat
 285 mg sodium

Macadamia Nut Torte

(No Wheat, Milk, Gluten)

___

1 jar (5–7 ounces) macadamia nuts
½ cup potato starch
1 teaspoon baking powder
6 large eggs, separated (at room temperature)
1 cup sugar
1 teaspoon vanilla extract

Preheat oven to 325°F. In a food processor fitted with the metal blade, process the nuts, potato starch, and baking powder until the nuts are finely chopped (10–15 pulses). Empty out onto a piece of wax paper. Process the egg yolks and sugar until thick and pale yellow, about 40 seconds, scraping the sides of the work bowl once during that time. Beat the egg whites in a large mixing bowl with an electric mixer, until stiff peaks form. Fold the yolk-and-sugar mixture into the beaten whites with a spatula. Sprinkle the nut-flour mixture on top and fold in gently, but thoroughly, along with the vanilla. Pour the batter into a 10-inch ungreased tube pan and bake until a cake tester or toothpick comes out clean, 35–40 minutes. Let cool in pan until room temperature. Run a knife around the inside edge carefully and remove the cake by inverting it onto a cake plate. Cover with plastic wrap until ready to serve. Dust with confectioners' sugar and serve with fresh fruit.

Makes 12 servings
One serving = 221   calories
              4 g   protein
             31 g   carbohydrates
              9 g   fat
           407 mg   sodium

◈

Baked Rice Pudding

(No Wheat, Gluten)

_____

1 cup cooked brown rice
1 teaspoon vanilla extract
¼ cup raisins
2 cups low-fat milk
3 tablespoons sugar
2 eggs

Preheat oven to 325°F. Combine all ingredients in bowl. Pour into lightly oiled casserole dish. Bake 45–50 minutes, or until knife inserted into center comes out clean.

Makes 4 servings
One serving = 118   calories
4 g   protein
21 g   carbohydrates
2 g   fat
301 mg   sodium

Oatmeal Apple Crisp

(No Wheat, Egg, Milk)

4 cups sliced cooking apples
1 tablespoon lemon juice
1 cup oatmeal
½ cup honey
1 teaspoon cinnamon
¼ cup margarine

Preheat oven to 375°F. Place apples in shallow baking dish. Sprinkle with lemon juice. Combine remaining ingredients; mix until crumbly. Sprinkle crumb mixture over apples. Bake 30 minutes or until apples are tender.

Makes 6 servings
One serving = 125   calories
             1 g   protein
          24 g   carbohydrates
            3 g   fat
      104 mg   sodium

⊷

Potato Starch Sponge Cake

(No Wheat, Milk, Gluten)

---

4 eggs, separated
1 cup sugar
1 tablespoon lemon juice
1 tablespoon grated lemon rind
½ cup potato starch flour
1 teaspoon baking powder

Preheat oven to 350°F. In a small bowl, beat whites until stiff, but not dry. In a separate bowl, beat egg yolks. Add sugar, lemon juice, and grated rind. Beat thoroughly. Stir in flour and baking powder. Beat until light yellow and smooth. Fold in beaten egg whites. Pour into ungreased tube pan. Bake 30–40 minutes. Invert pan to cool.

Makes 12 servings
One serving = 112 calories
　　　　　2 g protein
　　　　　22 g carbohydrates
　　　　　2 g fat
　　　197 mg sodium

Rice Cereal Crumb Crust

(No Wheat, Milk, Egg, Gluten)

---

1 cup crushed crisp rice cereal
¼ cup sugar
⅓ cup margarine, melted

Preheat oven to 375°F. Mix cereal crumbs, sugar, and margarine. Press firmly into bottom and sides of 9-inch pie pan. Bake 8 minutes until lightly browned. Crust may be refrigerated for 1 hour before filling instead of baking.

Makes 7 servings
One serving = 142   calories
2 g   protein
22 g   carbohydrates
6 g   fat
328 mg   sodium

Rice Flour Pie Crust

(No Wheat, Egg, Milk, Gluten)

¾ cup rice flour
1 teaspoon sugar
¼ teaspoon salt
⅓ cup margarine
2 tablespoons cold water

Preheat oven to 350°F. Stir together dry ingredients. Cut in margarine until pieces are size of peas. Add cold water a tablespoon at a time. Toss until a ball is formed. Roll dough to ⅛-inch thickness between two sheets of foil or waxed paper. Peel off top sheet and fit dough into 9-inch pie pan. Peel off other sheet. Prick dough with fork. Bake 15 minutes until brown.

Makes 7 servings
One serving = 118 calories
2 g protein
12 g carbohydrates
6 g fat
449 mg sodium

❧

Barley Pie Crust

(No Wheat, Milk, Egg)

1½ cups barley flour
1 teaspoon sugar
½ teaspoon salt
⅓ cup vegetable shortening
4 tablespoons cold water

Preheat oven to 350°F. Stir together all dry ingredients. Cut in shortening until pieces are size of peas. Add cold water a tablespoon at a time until a ball is formed. Roll dough to ⅛-inch thickness between 2 sheets of foil or waxed paper. Peel off top sheet and fit dough into 9-inch pie pan. Peel off top sheet. Trim edges of dough to fit pan. Prick with fork. Bake 15 minutes until brown.

Rice Crust Substitute 1¼ cup rice flour for barley flour. This crust can be pressed into pan instead of rolling.

Rye Crust Substitute 1½ cups rye flour for barley flour.

Makes 7 servings
One serving = 132　calories
2 g　protein
16 g　carbohydrates
7 g　fat
464 mg　sodium

ॐॐ

Spelt Pie Crust

(No Wheat, Milk, Egg)

---

3 tablespoons oil
2 tablespoons cool water
¼ teaspoon salt
1 cup plus 2 tablespoons spelt flour

Preheat oven to 375°F. Whisk oil, water, and salt together. Stir in the flour and mix only until evenly moistened. Press into a 9-inch pie plate. Bake crust 12 minutes. Fill when crust has cooled.

Makes 7 servings
One serving =   124   calories
             2 g   protein
          14 g   carbohydrates
           7 g   fat
     322 mg   sodium

❧

Coconut Crust

(No Wheat, Milk, Egg)

¼ cup margarine, melted
2 cups flake-type coconut

Preheat oven to 325°F. Thoroughly combine margarine and coconut. Press evenly into 9-inch pie pan. Bake 30–35 minutes until lightly browned.

Makes 7 servings
One serving = 121   calories
0 g   protein
3 g   carbohydrates
12 g   fat
291 mg   sodium

11

Cookies, Snacks, and Milk Alternatives

Barley Flour Brownies

(No Wheat, Egg)

---

2 cups barley flour
2 tablespoons potato starch
1 cup sugar
1 tablespoon baking powder
2 ounces unsweetened chocolate, melted
⅓ cup chopped nuts
¼ cup vegetable oil
¾ cup rice milk

Preheat oven to 350°F. Combine all ingredients in a mixing bowl. Pour batter into lightly oiled 8-inch square baking pan. Bake 30–35 minutes. Remove pan from oven and cool 5 minutes. Cut into squares.

Makes 18 squares
One square = 165   calories
            3 g   protein
           22 g   carbohydrates
            9 g   fat
          204 mg   sodium

Rye Raisin Bars

(No Wheat, Milk, Egg)

BARS

> 1 cup firmly packed brown sugar
> 1 cup water
> 3 tablespoons vegetable oil
> 1 teaspoon cinnamon
> 1 teaspoon nutmeg
> 1/4 teaspoon ground cloves
> 1/4 teaspoon salt
> 1 cup raisins
> 24 rye wafers rolled into crumbs
> 1/2 teaspoon baking soda

GLAZE

> 1 tablespoon warm water
> 1 teaspoon lemon juice
> 1 cup sifted confectioners' sugar

Preheat oven to 350°F. Place brown sugar, water, oil, spices, salt, and raisins in a medium saucepan. Bring the mixture to a boil and cook 5 minutes, stirring frequently. Remove from heat. Stir in rye wafers and baking soda. Pour into lightly oiled 8-inch square pan and bake 30 minutes. Combine ingredients for glaze. Spread evenly over the contents of the pan. Cool and cut into bars.

Makes 24 bars
One bar = 146   calories
              2 g   protein
             32 g   carbohydrates
              2 g   fat
           202 mg   sodium

❧

Apricot Squares

(No Wheat, Egg, Milk, Gluten)

1¼ *cups dried apricots, chopped*
1 *cup water*
1½ *cups rice flour*
2 *tablespoons tapioca starch*
2 *tablespoons brown sugar*
½ *teaspoon cinnamon*
⅓ *cup margarine*

Preheat oven to 350°F. Combine apricots and water in saucepan. Cook over low heat until mixture is thick. Puree in blender and set aside. Make crust by combining flour, starch, brown sugar, and cinnamon in mixing bowl. Cut in margarine until mixture resembles coarse cornmeal. Pack about two-thirds of crumble mixture into 9-inch square ungreased baking pan. Spread apricot mixture evenly over crust. Cover with remaining crumble mixture. Pack lightly. Bake 20 minutes. Cool; cut into squares.

Makes 16 squares
One square = 126   calories
             2 g   protein
            21 g   carbohydrates
             4 g   fat
           177 mg   sodium

❧

Rice Flour Brownies

(No Wheat, Egg, Milk, Gluten)

---

2 1-ounce squares unsweetened chocolate
¼ cup vegetable oil
¾ cup sugar
1 cup rice flour
1 teaspoon baking powder
2 tablespoons tapioca or potato starch
¼ teaspoon salt
1 teaspoon vanilla extract
½ cup water
½ cup chopped nuts

Preheat oven to 350°F. Melt chocolate, oil, and sugar in a small saucepan over low heat. Cool. In a separate bowl combine flour, baking powder, starch, and salt. Add chocolate mixture, vanilla, water, and nuts. Pour into an 8-inch square pan. Bake 25–30 minutes. Cool. Cut into squares.

Makes 16 brownies
One brownie = 163   calories
            2 g   protein
           23 g   carbohydrates
            9 g   fat
          221 mg   sodium

Applesauce Bars

(No Wheat, Milk, Gluten)

½ cup vegetable oil
½ cup sugar
1 egg
1½ cups rice flour
¼ cup soy flour or tapioca starch
¼ teaspoon salt
2 teaspoons baking powder
½ teaspoon baking soda
¼ teaspoon ground nutmeg
¼ teaspoon ground cloves
1 teaspoon ground cinnamon
1 cup applesauce
½ cup raisins
½ cup chopped nuts

Preheat oven to 375°F. Cream oil, sugar, and egg together. Stir in the remaining ingredients. Pour into lightly oiled 13″ × 9″ baking pan. Bake 20–25 minutes. Cool and cut into bars.

Makes 15 bars
One bar = 163   calories
           2 g   protein
          20 g   carbohydrates
          10 g   fat
         219 mg sodium

Minifruitcake Cookies

(No Wheat, Milk, Gluten)

1/4 cup vegetable oil
1/2 cup brown sugar, packed
1 egg
1 3/4 cups rice flour
1 tablespoon potato starch
1 teaspoon baking powder
1/2 teaspoon ground cinnamon
1/4 teaspoon ground nutmeg
1 1/2 teaspoons orange extract
3/4 cup (6 ounces) diced candied fruits
1/2 cup currants
1/2 cup chopped walnuts
1/4 cup apple juice

Preheat oven to 350°F. Cream together oil, brown sugar, and egg. Add rice flour, potato starch, baking powder, cinnamon, nutmeg, and orange extract. Mix well. Stir in candied fruits, currants, walnuts, and apple juice. Mix well. Drop by spoonfuls onto lightly oiled baking sheet. Bake 15–20 minutes or until browned. Cool on rack before storing.

Makes 30 cookies
One cookie = 144   calories
          2 g   protein
       26 g   carbohydrates
        4 g   fat
   188 mg   sodium

Oatmeal Applesauce Cookies

(No Wheat, Milk)

---

1 cup teff flour
1 cup quick rolled oats
½ cup date sugar
2 teaspoons baking powder
1 teaspoon ground cinnamon
¼ teaspoon ground nutmeg
¼ teaspoon ground cloves
½ cup currants
¼ cup honey
½ cup applesauce
1 egg
½ cup vegetable oil

Preheat oven to 375°F. Combine flour, oats, sugar, baking powder, and spices in a mixing bowl. Add the remaining ingredients and mix well. Drop by spoonfuls onto lightly oiled baking pan. Bake 10–15 minutes or until cookies are firm. Cool on rack.

Makes 36 cookies
One cookie = 118 calories
      2 g protein
      19 g carbohydrates
      4 g fat
      191 mg sodium

Rye Molasses Drop Cookies

(No Wheat, Milk, Egg)

½ cup milk-free margarine
½ cup sugar
½ cup molasses
2 cups rye flour
2 teaspoons baking powder
¼ teaspoon ground ginger
½ teaspoon nutmeg
½ cup applesauce
½ cup raisins

Preheat oven to 375°F. Lightly grease two baking sheets. Cream together shortening, sugar, and molasses. Sift together dry ingredients. Add dry ingredients alternately with applesauce to creamed mixture. Add raisins and stir to combine. Drop by rounded teaspoons onto baking sheets. Bake 10 minutes.

Makes 48 cookies
One cookie = 132   calories
            2 g   protein
         21 g   carbohydrates
          5 g   fat
    229 mg   sodium

Chocolate Chip Cookies

(No Wheat, Milk, Gluten)

⅓ *cup sugar*
⅓ *cup vegetable oil*
1 *egg*
⅔ *cup rice flour*
¼ *cup potato flour*
2 *teaspoons baking powder*
1 *teaspoon vanilla*
½ *cup chocolate chips*

Preheat oven to 375°F. Cream together sugar, oil, and egg. Add flours, baking powder, and vanilla. Add chocolate pieces. Beat to combine. Drop by spoonfuls onto lightly oiled baking sheet. Bake 10–12 minutes.

Makes 18 cookies
One cookie = 152 calories
         2 g protein
     23 g carbohydrates
      8 g fat
  191 mg sodium

Eggless Chocolate Chip Cookies

(No Wheat, Egg, Milk, Gluten)

⅓ cup soft margarine
⅓ cup sugar
¼ cup brown sugar
6 tablespoons water
⅔ cup soy flour
½ cup brown rice flour
3 tablespoons potato flour
3 teaspoons baking powder
¼ teaspoon salt
1 teaspoon vanilla
1 cup chocolate chips or carob pieces
½ cup chopped nuts

Preheat oven to 375°F. Cream together margarine, sugars, vanilla, and water. Blend in flours, baking powder, and salt. Beat until smooth. Stir in chocolate chips and nuts. Drop by spoonfuls onto lightly oiled cookie sheet. Bake 8–10 minutes.

Makes 36 cookies
Two cookies =　223　calories
　　　　　　　2 g　protein
　　　　　　29 g　carbohydrates
　　　　　　11 g　fat
　　　　206 mg　sodium

Teff Chocolate Chip Cookies

(No Egg, Milk)

1½ cups teff flour
½ cup tapioca flour
¾ cup sugar
1 tablespoon baking powder
½ cup water
⅓ cup vegetable oil
½ cup chocolate chips
½ cup chopped nuts

Preheat oven to 375°F. Combine all ingredients in mixing bowl. Mix well. Drop dough by spoonfuls onto lightly oiled baking sheet. Bake 10–15 minutes, or until browned.

Makes 24 cookies
One cookie = 171 calories
2 g protein
32 g carbohydrates
7 g fat
178 mg sodium

Spelt Chocolate Chip Cookies

(No Milk, Egg)

1½ cups spelt flour
½ cup tapioca flour
½ cup brown sugar
1 tablespoon baking powder
½ cup water
⅓ cup vegetable oil
½ cup chopped nuts
½ cup chocolate chips

Preheat oven to 375°F. Combine all ingredients in mixing bowl and mix well. Drop dough by spoonfuls onto lightly oiled baking sheets. Bake 10–15 minutes or until browned.

Makes 30 cookies
One cookie = 181 calories
          2 g   protein
      28 g   carbohydrates
       7 g   fat
  169 mg   sodium

❦

Millet Peanut Butter Cookies

(No Wheat, Milk)

½ cup peanut butter
¼ cup vegetable oil
⅓ cup brown sugar, packed
1 egg
1½ cups millet flour
2 teaspoons baking powder
¼ cup water

Preheat oven to 375°F. Cream together peanut butter, oil, brown sugar, and egg. Stir in flour, baking powder, and water. Beat well. Shape into walnut-size balls and place on lightly oiled cookie sheets. Flatten with fork. Bake 15–20 minutes.

Makes 36 cookies
One cookie = 130 calories
             2 g protein
            30 g carbohydrates
             5 g fat
           244 mg sodium

Peanut Butter Cookies

(No Wheat, Milk, Gluten)

1/3 cup margarine
1/2 cup peanut butter
1/2 cup brown sugar
1 teaspoon vanilla
1 egg
1/4 cup potato flour
1/4 cup rice polish
1/2 cup rice flour
1/2 teaspoon baking soda
2 teaspoons baking powder

Preheat oven to 375°F. Cream together margarine, peanut butter, brown sugar, vanilla, and egg. Stir in potato flour, rice polish, rice flour, baking soda, and baking powder. Beat until all ingredients are well mixed. Form into 36 pecan-size balls. Put on ungreased cookie sheets and flatten with fork. Bake 10 minutes.

Makes 36 cookies
One cookie = 147 calories
2 g protein
24 g carbohydrates
7 g fat
198 mg sodium

❧

Peanut Butter Balls

(No Wheat, Egg, Milk, Gluten)

½ cup peanut butter
2 tablespoons lemon juice
1 cup chopped dates or raisins

Mix peanut butter, lemon juice, and fruit. Form into ½-inch balls. Store in airtight container.

Makes 24 balls
One ball = 96   calories
1 g   protein
16 g   carbohydrates
4 g   fat
108 mg   sodium

Chocolate Peanut Butter Chewies

(No Wheat, Gluten)

4 ounces (4 squares) semisweet chocolate
¼ cup (½ stick) butter or margarine
½ cup peanut butter
1 cup granulated sugar
2 large eggs, lightly beaten
1 tablespoon unsweetened cocoa powder
1 teaspoon pure vanilla extract
¼ cup tapioca or rice flour

Preheat oven to 325°F. Combine chocolate, butter, and peanut butter in a medium saucepan. Cook over low heat, stirring often, until smooth. Remove from heat and stir in granulated sugar. Cool 1–2 minutes; add eggs, cocoa, and vanilla. Mix thoroughly. Stir in flour. Pour batter into an 8-inch square baking pan lined with aluminum foil. Bake until set, 35–40 minutes. Cool in pan 20 minutes. Carefully lift foil from pan and cool thoroughly. Freeze until firm. To serve, cut into squares or triangles. Store in airtight container or freeze for up to 2 weeks.

Makes 16 squares
One square = 169   calories
             2 g   protein
          28 g   carbohydrates
            7 g   fat
      119 mg   sodium

Barley Oatmeal Cookies

(No Wheat, Egg, Milk)

1½ *cups barley flour*
1 *cup quick oats*
¼ *cup tapioca flour*
½ *teaspoon ground cinnamon*
¼ *teaspoon ground nutmeg*
¼ *teaspoon ground ginger*
½ *cup maple syrup or honey*
½ *cup applesauce*
½ *cup raisins or currants*
⅓ *cup vegetable oil*
1 *tablespoon baking powder*

Preheat oven to 375°F. Combine all ingredients in mixing bowl. Beat well to blend. Drop by spoonfuls onto lightly oiled baking sheet. Bake 10–15 minutes or until browned.

Makes 36 cookies
One cookie = 166   calories
2 g   protein
29 g   carbohydrates
8 g   fat
189 mg   sodium

❧

Quinoa Raisin Cookies

(No Wheat, Egg, Milk)

1½ *cups quinoa flour*
½ *cup tapioca flour*
¾ *cup sugar*
1 *tablespoon baking powder*
½ *cup water*
⅓ *cup vegetable oil*
½ *cup raisins or currants*
½ *cup applesauce*
1 *teaspoon ground allspice*

Preheat oven to 375°F. Combine flours, sugar, and baking powder in mixing bowl. Add the remaining ingredients. Mix well. Drop by spoonfuls onto lightly oiled baking sheet. Bake 10–12 minutes until browned.

Makes 36 cookies
One cookie = 171   calories
              2 g   protein
             28 g   carbohydrates
              7 g   fat
            198 mg   sodium

≈⅍

Rye Orange Squares

(No Wheat, Egg, Milk)

1¾ *cups rye flour*
¼ *cup potato starch*
¾ *cup sugar*
1 *tablespoon baking powder*
½ *cup water or orange juice*
¼ *cup vegetable oil*
Grated peel of 1 orange
1 *teaspoon orange extract*

Preheat oven to 375°F. Combine all dry ingredients in mixing bowl. Stir to blend. Add the remaining ingredients. Stir well. Pour batter into lightly oiled 8-inch square baking pan. Bake 20–25 minutes. Cool. Cut into squares.

Makes 15 squares
One square = 161   calories
2 g   protein
26 g   carbohydrates
6 g   fat
176 mg   sodium

Quinoa Lemon Squares

(No Wheat, Milk)

2 cups quinoa flour
½ cup vegetable oil
¼ cup sugar
4 eggs
1 cup sugar
¼ cup arrowroot
1 teaspoon baking powder
¼ cup lemon juice
½ teaspoon lemon extract
Grated lemon peel
Powdered sugar

Preheat oven to 350°F. Using a fork, mix together quinoa flour, oil, and ¼ cup sugar. Pat mixture into bottom of 9″ × 13″ baking pan. Bake 20 minutes. Meanwhile beat eggs until light and fluffy. Stir in 1 cup sugar, arrowroot, baking powder, lemon juice, and lemon peel. Pour over crust. Bake 20–25 minutes longer. Cool; cut into bars. Sprinkle with powdered sugar before serving.

Makes 24 squares
One square = 162   calories
            2 g   protein
         25 g   carbohydrates
          7 g   fat
    188 mg   sodium

⌘

Raisin Spice Cookies

(No Wheat, Milk, Gluten)

½ cup sugar
½ cup vegetable oil
1 egg
1 cup rice flour
¼ cup potato flour
2 teaspoons baking powder
½ teaspoon baking soda
½ teaspoon ground cinnamon
¼ teaspoon ground nutmeg
½ cup raisins
½ cup chopped pecans

Preheat oven to 375°F. Cream together sugar, oil, and egg. Add rice flour, potato flour, baking powder, baking soda, cinnamon, and nutmeg. Mix well. Stir in raisins and pecans. Drop onto lightly oiled baking sheet. Bake 12–15 minutes.

Makes 24 cookies
One cookie = 174   calories
2 g   protein
25 g   carbohydrates
9 g   fat
186 mg   sodium

Fruitcake Cookies

(No Wheat, Milk, Gluten)

1 egg
½ cup vegetable oil
½ cup sugar
1 cup brown rice flour
2 tablespoons to ¼ cup potato flour
2 teaspoons baking powder
⅓ cup currants or raisins
⅓ cup chopped dates
⅓ cup chopped apricots
⅓ cup chopped walnuts
½ cup orange juice

Preheat oven to 375°F. Cream together egg, oil, and sugar. Add remaining ingredients. Mix well. Drop by spoonfuls onto lightly oiled baking sheet. Bake 10–15 minutes or until browned.

Makes 36 cookies
One cookie =   158   calories
                2 g   protein
               31 g   carbohydrates
                4 g   fat
              101 mg   sodium

⌇

Millet-Aplesauce Cookies

(No Wheat, Egg, Milk)

---

2 cups millet flour
1½ teaspoons baking powder
½ cup unsweetened applesauce
¾ cup apple juice concentrate, thawed
½ cup oil
1 cup milk-free unsweetened carob chips or
    chopped nuts (optional)

Preheat oven to 350°F. Mix flour and baking soda in a large bowl. Combine the applesauce, apple juice concentrate, and oil in a small bowl. Add the liquids to the flour mixture and stir just until mixed. Fold in the chips or nuts. Drop by heaping teaspoonfuls onto an ungreased baking sheet. Bake 15–20 minutes or until cookies begin to brown.

Makes about 36 cookies
One cookie = 111   calories
            2 g   protein
           19 g   carbohydrates
            3 g   fat
           87 mg sodium

❧

Orange Potato Flour Sponge Squares

(No Wheat, Milk, Gluten)

---

2 eggs, separated, egg whites stiffly beaten
½ cup sugar
¼ teaspoon salt
1 teaspoon orange extract
½ cup potato starch flour

Preheat oven to 325°F. Beat egg yolks and sugar together until thick and lemon-colored. Add salt, orange extract, and flour. Mix until smooth. Fold in stiffly beaten egg whites. Pour into lightly oiled 8-inch square pan. Bake 20–25 minutes until very lightly browned. Cut into squares.

Makes 16 squares
One square = 87   calories
             2 g   protein
            21 g   carbohydrates
             1 g   fat
           196 mg sodium

Amaranth Spice Cookies

(No Wheat, Egg, Milk)

1½ cups amaranth flour
2 tablespoons potato starch
2 teaspoons baking powder
½ cup vegetable oil
⅔ cup sugar
1 teaspoon ground cinnamon
¼ teaspoon ground cloves
¼ cup orange juice
Grated orange rind

Preheat oven to 375°F. Mix all ingredients in a medium mixing bowl. Blend well. Drop by spoonfuls onto lightly oiled baking sheet. Bake 10–15 minutes.

Makes 20 cookies
One cookie = 143 calories
2 g protein
23 g carbohydrates
6 g fat
179 mg sodium

৵

Coconut Macaroons

(No Wheat, Milk, Gluten)

---

1 3½-ounce can flaked coconut
4 egg whites, unbeaten
1 cup sugar
¼ cup potato starch flour
1 teaspoon almond extract

Preheat oven to 300°F. Lightly grease a baking sheet. Mix all ingredients together in saucepan and cook over medium heat until mixture is as thick as mashed potatoes (about 8 minutes), stirring constantly. Drop by teaspoons onto baking sheet. Bake 20 minutes.

Makes 36 cookies
One cookie = 86   calories
             1 g   protein
            17 g   carbohydrates
             3 g   fat
            97 mg sodium

❧

Marshmallow Crispies

(No Wheat, Gluten, Milk, Eggs)

---

2 tablespoon milk-free margarine
1 cup marshmallow creme or
    2 cups miniature marshmallows
3 cups crisp rice cereal

Melt margarine in a saucepan over low heat. Add marshmallow creme and heat approximately 5 minutes until melted. Remove from heat. Stir in cereal. Pour into lightly oiled 8-inch square pan. Pack firmly. Let stand until firm. Cut into 24 bars.

Makes 24 bars
One bar = 118   calories
        2 g   protein
       25 g   carbohydrates
        2 g   fat
      141 mg   sodium

Oatmeal Fruit Chews

(No Wheat, Milk, Egg)

1 cup chopped dried dates, figs, prunes, or
    apricots
¼ cup sugar
¼ cup plus 2 tablespoons water
2 tablespoons lemon juice
2 cups oatmeal
½ teaspoon baking soda
½ cup firmly packed brown sugar
½ cup shortening or margarine

Preheat oven to 350°F. Combine fruit, sugar, and water in a medium saucepan. Cook until smooth; add lemon juice. Cool. Combine oatmeal, baking soda, and brown sugar; cut in shortening. Take out one-third crumb mixture for topping. Add water to remainder. Pack dough into lightly oiled 8-inch pan. Spread fruit filling over and sprinkle with crumbs. Bake 30 minutes.

Makes 16 squares
One square = 165   calories
         2 g   protein
      33 g   carbohydrates
       5 g   fat
   119 mg   sodium

❧

Puffed Rice Balls

(No Wheat, Egg, Milk, Gluten)

---

2 tablespoons vegetable oil
½ cup chopped dates
¼ cup sugar
¼ cup chopped nuts
2 cups puffed rice cereal, crushed

Combine oil, dates, and sugar in a small saucepan. Cook about 4 minutes until mixture is thick. Stir in nuts and cereal. Mix well. Shape into walnut-sized balls.

Makes 18 balls
One ball = 118 calories
2 g protein
19 g carbohydrates
4 g fat
147 mg sodium

Rye Flour Bars

(No Wheat, Egg, Milk)

1¾ *cups rye flour*
1 *cup sugar*
1 *teaspoon baking powder*
½ *cup water*
3 *tablespoons vegetable oil*
1 *teaspoon vanilla extract*

Preheat oven to 350°F. Combine dry ingredients. Mix liquids together in a separate bowl, then stir into dry ingredients. Mix well. Pat the dough into oiled and floured 8-inch square pan. Bake 30–35 minutes. Cut immediately, then cool.

Makes 16 bars
One bar = 126 calories
2 g protein
27 g carbohydrates
2 g fat
116 mg sodium

🌿

Barley Cookies

(No Wheat, Milk)

½ cup shortening or margarine
1 cup sugar
2 eggs
2 cups barley flour
4 teaspoons baking powder
½ teaspoon salt
¼ cup orange, apple, or apricot juice

Preheat oven to 350°F. Cream shortening, sugar, and egg until light and fluffy. Sift together dry ingredients. Add alternately with juice. Drop by teaspoonfuls onto lightly oiled baking sheet. Bake 15 minutes until lightly browned.

Makes 36 cookies
One cookie = 138   calories
　　　　　　 2 g   protein
　　　　　　 26 g   carbohydrates
　　　　　　 4 g   fat
　　　　　　186 mg   sodium

≈⧉

Sugar Cookies

(No Wheat, Milk, Gluten)

¾ cup margarine
½ cup sugar
2 eggs
1 teaspoon vanilla extract
1 teaspoon liquid butter flavoring
2¼ cups rice flour
4 teaspoons baking powder
½ teaspoon salt

Preheat oven 375°F. Cream shortening, sugar, eggs, and flavorings until light and fluffy. Stir together dry ingredients in a separate bowl; add to creamed mixture. Mix well. Place dough on board lightly dusted with rice flour; roll to ⅛-inch thickness. Cut with small cookie cutters. Sprinkle with plain or colored sugar. Arrange cookies on lightly greased baking sheets. Bake 10 minutes until lightly browned.

Makes 60 cookies
One cookie = 92   calories
              1 g   protein
             19 g   carbohydrates
              2 g   fat
             44 mg sodium

≈❧

Barley Flour Sugar Cookies

(No Wheat, Milk, Egg)

2½ *cups barley flour*
½ *cup sugar*
1½ *teaspoons baking powder*
½ *cup vegetable oil*
½ *cup water or Nut Milk (See Index.)*
2 *teaspoons lemon extract*

Preheat oven to 350°F. Combine flour, sugar, and baking powder in mixing bowl. Add oil, water, and lemon extract. Mix well to moisten all flour. Press dough into ball. Roll dough onto floured surface to ¼-inch thick. Cut into shapes. Bake 15–20 minutes or until cookies are browned.

Makes 36 cookies
One serving = 139 calories
  2 g protein
  24 g carbohydrates
  4 g fat
  174 mg sodium

⊸✤

Pecan Turtle Cookies

(No Wheat, Egg, Gluten)

1½ cups margarine or butter
2 cups brown sugar, packed firm
1½ cups white rice flour
¼ cup tapioca flour
¼ cup potato starch flour
1 cup pecans, whole or chopped
12 ounces milk chocolate chips

Preheat oven to 350°F. Combine ½ cup margarine, 1 cup brown sugar, white rice flour, tapioca flour, and potato flour in mixing bowl. Beat until particles are fine. The mixture will look dry. Pat firmly into a 9″ × 13″ pan. Sprinkle pecans evenly over the unbaked crust.

In a saucepan, combine the remaining brown sugar and margarine. Cook over medium heat, stirring constantly, until entire surface of mixture begins to boil. Boil ½ minute, stirring constantly. Pour evenly over pecans and crust. Bake 18–20 minutes. Remove from oven and immediately sprinkle with chocolate chips. Allow chips to melt slightly, then swirl chips with a toothpick. Leave some chips nearly whole for a marbled effect. Let cookies continue to cool, but cut into bars before cookies are cold. Chill in refrigerator to finish setting the chocolate.

Makes 24 cookies
One cookie = 212   calories
              2 g   protein
             34 g   carbohydrates
             11 g   fat
             98 mg   sodium

&⅞

Chocolate Pecan Amaranth Brownies

(No Wheat, Egg, Milk)

---

2 cups amaranth flour
1 tablespoon baking powder
¼ cup arrowroot
⅔ cup sugar
½ cup cocoa
½ cup vegetable oil
¾ cup rice beverage or water
½ cup finely chopped pecans

Preheat oven to 375°F. Stir together all ingredients. Beat well. Pour batter into an oiled 8-inch square pan. Bake 25–30 minutes. Cool. Dust with confectioners' sugar.

Makes 9 brownies
One brownie = 164   calories
           2 g   protein
      29 g   carbohydrates
        7 g   fat
  127 mg   sodium

Rice Flour Lemon Squares

(No Wheat, Milk, Gluten)

⅓ cup margarine
3 tablespoons powdered sugar
1 cup brown rice flour
1½ teaspoons baking powder
½ cup sugar
2 eggs
2 teaspoons lemon rind
2 teaspoons lemon juice
2 teaspoons rice polish

Preheat oven to 350°F. Cream margarine and powdered sugar in a medium bowl. Blend in flour and press into an 8-inch square pan. Bake 20 minutes. Combine rest of ingredients and pour over baked crust. Bake 20 minutes longer. Remove the pan from the oven and allow to cool 30 minutes. Cut into squares.

Makes 16 squares
One square = 148   calories
             3 g   protein
            26 g   carbohydrates
             4 g   fat
           124 mg sodium

Barley Banana Spice Bars

(No Wheat, Egg, Milk)

---

2 very ripe bananas, cut into pieces
¼ cup vegetable oil
¾ cup sugar
2 cups barley flour
3 tablespoons arrowroot powder
1 teaspoon ground cinnamon
¼ teaspoon ground nutmeg
⅛ teaspoon ground cloves
Powdered sugar

Preheat oven to 375°F. Cream together bananas, oil, and sugar. Add the remaining ingredients. Mix well. Spoon batter into lightly oiled 8-inch square baking pan. Bake 20–25 minutes or until brown. Cool 30 minutes before cutting into bars. Top with sprinkling of powdered sugar before serving.

Makes 9 bars
One bar = 138   calories
            2 g   protein
           28 g   carbohydrates
            3 g   fat
          87 mg   sodium

Lemon Oatmeal Squares

(No Wheat)

2 cups rolled oats
¾ cup butter or margarine
1¼ cups sugar
4 eggs
¼ cup arrowroot
1 teaspoon baking powder
¼ cup lemon juice
Grated rind of 1 lemon
Ground nuts (optional)

Preheat oven to 350°F. Mix together oats, margarine, and ¼ cup sugar with pastry blender. Pat mixture into the bottom of a 9″ × 13″ baking pan. Bake 20 minutes. As the oatmeal mixture is baking, beat eggs until light and fluffy. Stir together 1 cup sugar, arrowroot, and baking powder. Add this to the eggs. Blend in lemon juice and rind. Pour over oatmeal mixture. Bake 25 minutes longer. Allow to cool; then cut into bars. Sprinkle with ground nuts, if desired.

Makes 32 squares
One square = 178   calories
            3 g   protein
         32 g   carbohydrates
          6 g   fat
      164 mg   sodium

≈⅄

Oatmeal Honey Bars

(No Wheat, Milk, Egg)

½ cup margarine
1 cup honey
2 cups oatmeal
¼ teaspoon salt
2 teaspoons baking powder

Preheat oven to 350°F. Combine butter and honey in a saucepan; cook and stir until butter is melted. Stir in remaining ingredients. Mix well. Pour into lightly oiled 8″ × 8″ × 2″ baking pan. Bake 20–25 minutes. Cool thoroughly. Cut into bars.

Makes 24 bars
One bar = 152 calories
2 g protein
29 g carbohydrates
4 g fat
176 mg sodium

Rice Delight

(No Wheat, Egg, Milk, Gluten)

½ cup uncooked rice
1 tablespoon honey or sugar
3 cups apple or orange juice
Dash of cinnamon
¼ cup raisins

Combine all ingredients in saucepan. Cook over low heat until rice is tender—about 1 hour—stirring occasionally to prevent sticking. Serve warm or cold.

Makes 4 servings
One serving =   94   calories
                2 g   protein
               22 g   carbohydrates
                0 g   fat
               74 mg sodium

Banana-Orange Tapioca

(No Wheat, Egg, Milk, Gluten)

¼ cup sugar
3 tablespoons minute tapioca
2 cups orange juice
2 teaspoons lemon juice
2 ripe bananas

Combine sugar and tapioca in saucepan. Add orange juice. Let stand 5 minutes. Cook and stir over medium heat until mixture comes to a boil. Remove from heat and stir in lemon juice. Cool, stirring once after 20 minutes. Chill. Top with sliced bananas.

Makes 5 servings
One serving = 58   calories
1 g   protein
12 g   carbohydrates
1 g   fat
87 mg   sodium

Amaranth Granola

(No Wheat, Egg, Milk)

1 cup amaranth flour
2 tablespoons carob powder
1/2 cup coarsely chopped pecans or other nuts
2 tablespoons sesame seeds
1/4 teaspoon salt
2 tablespoons vegetable oil
4 tablespoons maple syrup or molasses
4 tablespoons boiling water

Preheat oven to 250°F. Mix amaranth, carob powder, nuts, sesame seeds, and salt in a mixing bowl. In a small bowl or cup, mix the oil, maple syrup, and boiling water. Stir rapidly; then pour over the dry ingredients and mix well. Crumble the lumps. Cut through the mixture several times with a table knife until the particles are about the size of peas. Spread the mixture evenly on an oiled baking sheet with edges. Bake 30 minutes. Remove from oven and stir. Turn the oven off and allow granola mixture to cool in oven 1–2 hours. Store in a tightly sealed jar.

Makes 8 servings
One serving = 137 calories
            3 g protein
           18 g carbohydrates
            5 g fat
          203 mg sodium

❧

Crunchy Granola

(No Wheat, Egg, Milk, Gluten)

---

1 cup cooked brown rice
1 cup peanuts
1 cup shredded coconut
2 tablespoons sesame seeds
1 cup chopped nuts
¼ cup soy milk or apple juice
½ cup cream of rice cereal, uncooked
⅓ cup brown sugar
¼ cup vegetable oil

Preheat oven to 250°F. Combine all ingredients except oil on a baking sheet and mix with wooden spoon. Pour oil over mixture and toss lightly. Bake 1½ hours or until mixture is brown and dry. Stir mixture every 10–15 minutes during baking to toast evenly. Store in a tightly sealed container. Use as cereal or snack. This cereal can be stored on the pantry shelf if used within 2–3 weeks.

Makes 8 servings
One serving = 229 calories
4 g protein
33 g carbohydrates
11 g fat
206 mg sodium

Soy Rice Granola

(No Wheat, Egg, Milk, Gluten)

2/3 cup cream of rice
1 cup brown rice flour
1/2 cup rice polish
1/2 cup soy flour
1 cup soy flakes
1 cup unsweetened shredded coconut
1/4 cup sesame seeds
1 cup chopped pecans
1/3 cup brown sugar
3/4 cup water
1/4 cup vegetable oil

Preheat oven to 200°F. Combine all ingredients except water and oil on baking sheet. Drizzle on water and oil. Run mixture through hands to moisten. Toast 45–55 minutes. Cool and store in airtight container.

Makes 10 servings
One serving =   240   calories
                4 g   protein
           29 g   carbohydrates
           12 g   fat
     219 mg   sodium

🌿

Cereal Snack Mix

(No Wheat, Egg, Milk, Gluten)

---

4 cups toasted rice square cereal
2 cups puffed rice cereal
3 teaspoons margarine, melted
¼ teaspoon curry powder
½ teaspoon garlic powder
3 tablespoons sunflower kernels

Preheat oven to 350°F. Measure cereals into a large bowl. Pour on margarine, curry powder, and garlic powder. Toss to combine. Add sunflower kernels. Place mixture on baking sheet and toast in oven 10–15 minutes. Cool. Store in airtight container.

Makes 12 servings
One serving = 137   calories
            3 g   protein
      26 g   carbohydrates
            3 g   fat
   164 mg   sodium

Trail Mix

(No Wheat, Egg, Milk, Gluten)

½ cup unsalted peanuts
⅓ cup shredded unsweetened coconut
½ cup pecan halves
2 tablespoons sesame seeds
½ cup raisins
½ cup snipped apricots

In preheated 350°F oven, toast peanuts, coconut, pecans, and sesame seeds on a baking sheet until lightly browned (about 10–12 minutes). Cool and add dried fruit. Store in an airtight container.

Makes 5 servings
One serving =   164   calories
                   3 g   protein
                  29 g   carbohydrates
                   7 g   fat
                 139 mg   sodium

Milk Alternatives

Nut milk can be used for cereals, sauces, puddings, and as a milk replacement in recipes.

Almond Milk
1 cup pure water
4 tablespoons ground almonds

Brazil Nut Milk
1 cup pure water
4 tablespoons ground Brazil nuts

Cashew Nut Milk
1 cup pure water
4 tablespoons ground cashew nuts

Pecan Milk
1 cup pure water
4 tablespoons ground pecans

Sesame Milk
1 cup pure water
¼ cup sesame seeds

Walnut Milk
1 cup pure water
4 tablespoons ground walnuts

Blend well in blender or food processor. Strain to remove hulls or chunks (optional). Refrigerate up to three days.

Makes 1 cup
One serving = 175 calories
4 g protein
6 g carbohydrates
16 g fat
0 g sodium

12

Pizza Crusts

Rice Flour Pizza Crust

(No Wheat, Egg, Milk, Gluten)

---

1 cup brown rice flour
1 teaspoon sugar
1 package (1 tablespoon) dry yeast
⅓ cup warm (105°–110°F) water
1 tablespoon vegetable oil

Preheat oven to 400°F. Combine flour and sugar in a bowl. Dissolve yeast in water and stir until dissolved. Add yeast to flour along with oil. Mix well. Pat dough onto oiled baking sheet or pizza pan, keeping fingers lightly oiled to allow for even spreading. Use pizza sauce and topping of choice. Bake 20–25 minutes or until browned.

Makes 4 servings
One serving
(without topping) = 86   calories
                 1 g   protein
              12 g   carbohydrates
              4 g   fat
       142 mg   sodium

❧

Spelt Flour Pizza Crust

(No Wheat, Egg, Milk)

3½ cups spelt flour
1 tablespoon baking powder
½ teaspoon salt
⅓ cup vegetable oil
1¼ cups water

Preheat oven to 400°F. Combine flour, baking powder, and salt in a mixing bowl. Stir in oil and water. Mix well. With oiled hands pat into an oiled 12-inch pizza pan. Use pizza sauce and topping of choice. Bake 20–25 minutes or until browned.

Makes 8 servings
One serving (without topping) = 178   calories
2 g   protein
18 g   carbohydrates
12 g   fat
413 mg   sodium

⊷⅍

Amaranth Pizza Crust

(No Wheat, Egg, Milk)

3 cups amaranth flour
½ cup arrowroot
1 tablespoon baking powder
½ teaspoon salt
⅓ cup vegetable oil
1½ cups water

Preheat oven to 400°F. Combine flour, arrowroot, baking powder, and salt in a mixing bowl. Stir in oil and water. Mix well. With oiled hands pat into oiled 12-inch pizza pan. Use pizza sauce and topping of choice Bake 20–25 minutes or until browned.

Makes 8 servings
One serving (without topping) = 210   calories
3 g   protein
19 g   carbohydrates
14 g   fat
467 mg   sodium

❧

Rye Pizza Crust

(No Wheat, Egg, Milk)

---

3 cups rye flour
1 tablespoon baking powder
½ teaspoon salt
⅓ cup vegetable oil
1¼ cups water

Preheat oven to 400°F. Combine flour, baking powder, and salt in mixing bowl. Stir in oil and water. Mix well. With oiled hands pat into oiled 12-inch pizza pan. Use pizza sauce and topping of choice. Bake 20–25 minutes or until browned.

Makes 8 servings
One serving (without topping) = 208 calories
                                  1 g protein
                                 19 g carbohydrates
                                 13 g fat
                                437 mg sodium

❦

Quinoa Pizza Crust

(No Wheat, Egg, Milk)

---

3 cups quinoa flour
½ cup arrowroot
1 tablespoon baking powder
½ teaspoon salt
⅓ cup vegetable oil
1½ cups water

Preheat oven to 400°F. Combine flour, arrowroot, baking powder, and salt in a mixing bowl. Stir in oil and water. Mix well. With oiled hands pat into oiled 12-inch pizza pan. Use pizza sauce and topping of choice. Bake 20–25 minutes or until browned.

Makes 8 servings
One serving (without topping) = 209   calories
3 g   protein
20 g   carbohydrates
13 g   fat
457 mg   sodium

Appendix A

Food Allergy Terms and Definitions

acorn (Quercus prinus, Q. Emoroyi, Q. lobata). A nut that can be ground into a flour. It does not bind as well as wheat flour, but its nutty flavor makes it an excellent choice in chocolate and spice products. Also good for cookie and pancake recipes. You can gather dry acorns, shell, and toast for 2 minutes in a 350°F oven before grinding in a food processor to medium-coarse texture.

aflatoxin Produced by molds, this type of toxin has been shown to have a carcinogenic effect in animal experiments.

allergen Any substance that causes a state of sensitivity. The most common allergens are dusts, pollens, fungi, smoke, perfumes, odors of plastics, and foods such as wheat, gluten, eggs, milk, and chocolate.

allergic rhinitis Inflammation of nasal membranes due to sensitivity to an allergen.

allergy Acquired hypersensitivity to a substance (allergen) that does not normally cause a reaction. The reaction is due to the release of histamine from injured cells. An allergy may occur the second time a person is exposed to a particular allergen, or may not occur until years later when repeated exposures have produced sufficient antibodies.

almond (Prunus amygdalus) A nut that works well in breads, pastries, and cakes. It can be used in the form of coarse bits or as a flour and is an excellent addition to white or brown rice breads. The use of almond in rice bread makes a very good taste difference.

amaranth (Amaranthas candatas) A grain that is also commonly referred to as pigweed or tumbleweed. Amaranth flour originated with the Aztecs and makes smooth-textured baked goods. Not gluten free. Not recommended for use by people with celiac disease and dermatitis herpetiformis.

anaphylactic shock Severe allergic hypersensitivity reaction that could cause death if emergency treatment is not given. Symptoms vary from person to person, but can range from swollen tongue and lips to closed esophagus or cardiac arrest.

antibody Also called immunoglobulin. A large protein created by the body's immune system in response to an antigen.

antigen Substance that causes the formation of antibodies that interact specifically with it. An antigen may be introduced into the body by food or air particles, or it may be formed within the body.

arrowroot (maranta arundinacea) A tropical American plant with large leaves, white flowers, and starch roots. The starch made from the roots is typically used as a thickening agent and blends well with other flours.

arthralgia Pain in a joint or joints sometimes related to food allergies.

artichokes (articiocco) The flower head of a thistle-like plant that may be cooked and eaten as a vegetable. The dried artichoke may be ground into flour. It is an excellent addition to rice-potato-tapioca flour combinations for breads and coffee cakes.

azo dye A common food additive that may cause food sensitivities.

barley (hordeum vulgare) One of agriculture's oldest grains, often used in flavorings, colorings, malt, and as a flavor enhancer. It may be used as a part of hydrolyzed plant protein (HPP). Some food chemists indicate that it may also be a part of hydrolyzed vegetable protein (HVP) as an extender. Can be ground into flour or eaten cooked as a whole grain.

bean flour One of a family of basic protein flours available in health-food stores. They can easily be milled at home. Depending on taste preferences, they are excellent additions for bread and rolls. They each contribute to hardness in the product, so egg white and cottage cheese need to be added as softeners. They are common additions to gravies, meatloaf, soups, and sauces. Included with this listing of basic protein crops are the following: adzuki beans, asparagus beans, chickpeas, cowitch (the Florida velvet bean), cowpeas, groundnuts (peanuts), horse beans, hyancinth beans, kidney beans, lentils, lima beans, mung beans, peas, pigeon peas, ram mungs, scarlet runner beans, sievas, tepary beans.

buckwheat (Fagopyrum esculentum) A grain that is available as whole groats, cereal, and flour. Not gluten free. Not recommended for use by people with celiac disease and dermatitis herpetiformis.

bulgur Sometimes referred to as bulghur in recipes, this is a form of wheat. It is frequently available as a parboiled, soaked product which has then been dried. It may be available as wheat nuts. Bulgar and/or wheat in its natural state may be ground with carob and soybeans and used in breads and baked goods. Not gluten free. Not recommended for use by people with celiac disease and dermatitis herpetiformis.

carob (cara coa) A plant that is usually used as a replacement for chocolate. Those who are sensitive to soybeans and/or peanuts should not use carob since it is also a legume.

carrageenan (chondrus crispus or gigartina mammillosa) Obtained from seaweed and used as a substitute for some antigen products and as a thickening agent for such products as ice cream, jelly, and infant formula.

cassava Also called tapioca, yuca, manioc, mandioca, and aipim, a root that makes an excellent thickener for soups and gravies. It works best when ground into a fine flour consistency and incorporated into cookies and quick breads like pancakes and muffins.

celiac-sprue disease Also called gluten enteropathy. A syndrome that causes poor absorption of nutrients through the intestine. It requires a gluten-free diet.

corn flour (zea mays) A smooth flour that can be milled from the entire kernel of corn. It can also be blended with cornmeal and small amounts of other flours to make cornbread and cornmeal mush. Freeze corn products to avoid molds.

cornmeal Kernels of corn ground more coarsely than corn flour or cornstarch.

dermatitis herpetiformis Skin disorder characterized by an itchy rash caused by poor absorption of nutrients due to atrophy of the villi in the small intestine.

desensitization Prevention of allergic reaction or anaphylactic shock attained by receiving repeated doses of the sensitizing substance in too low a dose to cause a reaction.

dextrin A carbohydrate formed as an intermediate product in the digestion of starch.

eczema Inflammation of the skin with scales, crusts, or scabs, with or without watery discharge. Allergens aggravate the condition.

egg sensitivities Eggs are the second most common food allergy in infants and children. Egg whites are usually considered the major cause of the allergy.

flax (usitatissimum linn) A grain that is not usually seen as allergenic. It is typically listed as flaxseed or flaxseed oil on labels and may be listed as fiber in bulking agents and in high fiber foods. Some people who use it daily as a bowel agent may develop a sensitivity to it.

food additives Compounds that are added to food for color, preservation, or other reasons. The pharmacological effects of these chemicals are important to consider in asthma and food allergies.

food families Groups of foods from the same biological family. If someone is sensitive to one member of a food family, there is a possibility that other members of that food family may also be a source of irritation. *See* Appendix B.

food sensitivity, **food allergy**, and **food intolerance** Terms used interchangeably to refer to adverse reactions to food.

fruit sensitivities Reactions to fruits such as bananas and melons, often causing problems only during ragweed pollen season.

gastroenterologist A physician specializing in gastrointestinal disorders and diseases which may involve the digestive tract, liver, pancreas, and gallbladder.

gliaden A simple protein extracted from gluten in wheat or rye. A common allergen. *See* gluten.

gliadin-free diet *See* gluten-free diet.

gluten An elastic protein substance found in wheat and certain other grain flours. It helps dough stick together. A common allergen.

gluten enteropathy *See* celiac-sprue disease.

gluten-free diet Diet that avoids grains that contain gluten or gliadin, such as wheat. Recommended for people with celiac-sprue disease and dermatitis herpetiformis.

gluten-free flour blend A blend of gluten-free flours that can be used in place of wheat flour in recipes. It is made of 6 parts rice flour, 2 parts potato starch, and 1 cup tapioca flour.

histamine A substance normally present in the body but released at high levels from injured cells during an allergic reaction. Histamine increases digestive acids and capillary and muscle changes resulting in headaches, blood pressure changes, and skin reactions.

histamine foods Also called histamine releasers. Foods or chemicals that cause food-sensitivity symptoms. Certain foods already contain high levels of histamines, including: cheeses, spinach, eggplant, tomatoes, chicken livers, wines, tuna fish, strawberries, shellfish, egg whites, chocolate, and pineapple.

IgE Acronym used for immunoglobulin gamma E. A substance produced by cells in the lining of the lungs and intestines. High IgE antibody reactions are frequently found in people with allergic diseases.

IgG Acronym used for immunoglobulin gamma G. The principal immunoglobulin in human fluids. It is important in producing prebirth immunity in an infant because it crosses the placental barrier.

immune response Reaction of the body to substances that are foreign or interpreted by the body as foreign.

immunoassay A lab test that measures the protein and protein-bound molecules associated with an antigen or allergic reaction.

immunoglobulin *See* antibody.

intestinal dysbiosis The state of disordered ecology in the digestive tract that can cause disease.

intestinal permeability Also called leaky gut syndrome. Refers to a condition in which the spaces between cells in the gut are too far apart, causing the gut wall to leak substances into the bloodstream where they do not belong. These substances can cause food-allergy symptoms.

kamut (triticum polinicum) Also called pasta wheat or King Tut's wheat. A grain that makes tasty cookies, quick breads, and cakes. Not gluten free. Not recommended for use by people with celiac disease and dermatitis herpetiformis.

lactase An enzyme that is needed to digest lactose.

lactose A sugar present in milk. A common allergen.

leaky gut syndrome. *See* intestinal permeability.

malanga A root closely related to taro root, which is used to make poi (a cooked paste) in Polynesian countries. Malanga and taro root are in the arum family and frequently called Japanese potatoes. Malanga flour is used in cookies, quick breads, dumplings, and pasta. It is considered very hypoallergenic and easy to digest.

malt A grain product made from sprouted barley and the hydrolyzed starch of other grains. Malt is frequently used to add sweetness to prepared foods and is commonly found in ales, all-purpose flour, baby cereals, baby crackers, barbecue sauce, carob candy, beer, breakfast cereals, granolas, canned and dried soups, caramel flavoring, condiments, enriched bread, salad dressings, frozen dinners, lagers, malt liquor, maltodextrins, meat sauces, Ovaltine, Postum, processed meats, rye bread, bourbon, and whiskey. Not gluten free. Not recommended for use by people with celiac disease and dermatitis herpetiformis.

mast cell reactivity A large cell in connective tissue which can lead to the release of histamine and serotonin during inflammation and allergic response.

milk allergy A sensitivity to lactose, the protein in milk. Milk allergy is considered one of the most common food sensitivities among infants and children under age three. Requires a lactose-free diet.

millet A cereal grain available in a wide range of varieties. Common millets available in health-food stores include African millet, Italian millet, broomcorn millet, pearl millet, spiked millet, several German millets, and a number of hybrids from North Dakota and Canada. Not gluten free. Not recommended for use by people with celiac disease and dermatitis herpetiformis.

monosodium glutamate (MSG) A white substance used to enhance the flavor of foods and sold under various brand names such as Accent. When MSG is ingested in large amounts, those who are sensitive to it have reported chest pains, facial pressure, headaches, and excessive sweating. These symptoms have frequently been called Chinese restaurant syndrome because MSG is often used in Chinese dishes.

nut milk A milk-like liquid made from nuts or seeds that can be used on cereals, puddings, and in recipes as a milk replacement. *See* Index.

oats (Avena stativa) A cereal grain that is available in many varieties. Oats are best used in cereal, cookies, and quick breads. Not gluten free. Not recommended for use by people with celiac disease and dermatitis herpetiformis.

pea flour *See* bean flour.

potato (solanum tuberosum) A tuber that is eaten whole or ground into starch or flour. Those who are sulfite-sensitive should avoid commercially prepared potato products, because sulfites are used in processing to keep potatoes from turning brown. Those who are gluten-sensitive need to be aware that many commercially prepared french fries are packed in wheat flour that is used as a packaging agent and to increase browning during cooking.

potato flour Made from whole dried and ground potato. It allows batters to hold together and smooths the texture. This is *not* the same as *potato starch*. Do not substitute for potato starch in any recipe. Only small amounts are needed to smooth texture. Use 1 tablespoon potato flour per 1–2 cups rice flour or 1 teaspoon potato flour to ½ cup rice flour.

potato starch flour A highly milled product with a consistency similar to cornstarch that can be purchased at most supermarkets. It is *not* interchangeable with potato flour. Suggested use: for every cup of flour in the recipe, substitute ½ cup rice flour and ½ cup potato starch flour.

quinoa Pronounced KEEN-wa. A cereal grain from Peru, in the Goosefoot family, it is usually cooked and eaten like oatmeal. The flour has a nutty taste and can be made into cookies, pasta, quick breads, and dumplings. Not gluten free. Not recommended for use by people with celiac disease and dermatitis herpetiformis.

rhinitis Inflammation of the nasal membranes.

rice flour (oryza zativa) A white starch flour that can be labeled as white rice flour, brown rice flour, sweet rice flour, or wild rice flour. It has a tendency to give baked products a dry, grainy texture. Rice has a bland flavor that works best when combined with other gluten-free flours, especially potato starch flour. Sweet rice flour contains more starch than the brown and white rice flours and works well as a thickener because it holds a lot of moisture. Sweet rice is best used for sauces and gravies and can be found in Asian food stores. Wild rice (oryza fatua and oryza spontanea) is nutty tasting. It is grown in Minnesota, Wisconsin, and areas of Canada.

rye (secale cereale) A grain that works well when ground into a flour and combined with wheat to make bakery products. Not gluten free. Not recommended for use by people with celiac disease and dermatitis herpetiformis.

rye buckwheat (Fagopyrum tataricum) A grain that is not commonly available but may add variety to the diet as cooked cereal grain. Not gluten free. Not recommended for use by people with celiac disease and dermatitis herpetiformis.

sago (palm metroxylon sagus) A flour that is slightly gray in color and tastes rather bland, but can be used in baking. It is good in pastry—especially pizza dough—or in recipes with strong seasoning. It can be used for crumb toppings and in puddings.

semolina A type of wheat. The larger hard kernels of wheat that are sifted out in the flour milling process. Not gluten free. Not recommended for use by people with celiac disease and dermatitis herpetiformis.

sesame Seeds—used either whole, coarse ground, or as flour—that make an excellent addition to cookies and breads.

sorghum (sorgo, soreg, or L. syricus) Historically referred to as Syrian grass. Sorghum refers to a number of related cereal grasses with sweet juicy stalks grown for grain and syrups.

soy or **soya flour** (glycine max) A heavy flour made from ground soybeans with a strong, distinctive nut flavor that should be used in combination with other flours. It has a high protein and fat content and is best used in combination with other flours. It can be used in double chocolate cakes, spice cakes, and in cinnamon and pumpkin breads in which the flavor can be masked. It can add needed moisture to an otherwise dry recipe. Suggested use: If recipe calls for 2 cups flour, use 1 cup rice flour, ¾ cup potato starch flour, and ¼ cup soy flour.

spelt (triticum spelta) Also called dinkle. A nonhybridized wheat that has been grown in the Middle East for more than 9,000 years and is identified in some sources as manna. Like millet, spelt has evolved into many varieties. It is an excellent bread flour with unique gluten solubility, which makes for fine baked goods. Some people with wheat sensitivity can tolerate spelt since it is easy to digest. Not gluten free. Not recommended for use by people with celiac disease and dermatitis herpetiformis.

sulfite-free diet A diet free of many food additives. Recommended for people with asthma and sulfite sensitivity.

sulfites Found in many food additives, sulfites are a major cause of food sensitivity. They are widely used as a preservative in drugs and food, and as a bleaching agent in breads and bakery products.

sunflower seed A seed that may be eaten whole or ground fine and added to flour combinations.

sweet rice flour (also called sticky rice flour) *See* rice flour.

tapioca flour Made from cassava root, it can be used in pancake and waffle recipes to give them a light texture. Suggested use: $\frac{1}{4}$–$\frac{1}{2}$ cup of tapioca flour plus 1 cup of rice flour replaces 1 cup of wheat flour.

tartrazine A coal tar dye that can cause food- and drug-sensitivity problems. Many yellow-colored foods and foods with fruit flavors have tartrazine.

teff (eragrositis teff) Also called teff grass. Believed to have originated in Ethiopia as a wild grass that was eventually cultivated by Egyptians before 3000 B.C. Teff is the smallest grain in the world and is used to make the Ethiopian staple bread, injera. It can be used in cookies, quick breads, and cake recipes. Not gluten free. Not recommended for use by people with celiac disease and dermatitis herpetiformis.

triticale (x triticosecale) A hybrid grain combination of rye and wheat. Not gluten free. Not recommended for use by people with celiac disease and dermatitis herpetiformis.

urticaria Also called hives. Skin reaction caused from food, drugs, or insect bites. A sudden eruption of red bumps with intense itching is characteristic of this allergic response.

wheat (triticum aestivum) Also called common wheat. A common cereal grass crop that is found in many varieties. Contains gluten, a common allergen.

wheat-free diet Recommended for those who experience food-sensitivity symptoms from eating foods containing wheat such as bread, cake, pancakes, and cookies. *See also* gluten-free diet.

xanthan gum Made using the bacteria, Xanthomonas Compestris, to ferment corn sugar. It is used commercially to keep ingredients in suspension in salad dressings, pie fillings, gravies, and sauces, and in ice cream to give a smoother texture. Suggested use: 1 teaspoon per 1 cup flour.

yeast-free diet Recommended for those with yeast sensitivity and chronic yeast disorders of the gastrointestinal, urinary, or genital tract. (See "Yeast-Free and Mold-Free Diet" on page 77.)

Appendix B

Food Family Indexes

Food families can be used as a reference. If you react to more than two members of the same food family, there is a possibility that other members of that family may also be a source of irritation; although this is not always the case. Avoid these additional foods if symptoms continue.

Simple Food Family Index

This is the basic food family index used by many clinical ecologists to recommend menu and diet restrictions. It provides a basic outline of what foods have similar chemical and biological compounds and may produce similar allergic reactions.

Food Family	Related Foods
Banana/Musaceae	Arrowroot, plantains
Bass	Butterfish, cobia, crappie, croaker, drum fish, grouper, grunt, perch, red snapper, rockfish, sauger, sheephead, white perch, yellow bass
Bovine	Beef, bison, buffalo, calf, goat, lamb, ox, sheep, veal
Chocolate/ Theobromine/ Stericuliaceae	Chocolate, cocoa, cola, cola nut, gum karaya, theobromine
Citrus/Rutaceae	Angostura, calamondin, citron, grapefruit, kumquat, lemon, lime, mandarin, murcot, oranges, pomelo, satsuma, shaddock, tangerine, tangelo, ugly fruit

Codfish	coalfish, cod, cusk, haddock, hake, hoki, pollack, scrod, whiting
Composite/ Compositae	Artichoke, bibb lettuce, chamomile, chicory, dandelion, endive, escarole, Jerusalem artichoke, lettuce, oyster plant, romaine lettuce, safflower, salsify, stevia, sunflower seeds, tarragon, yarrow
Crustacean/Crustacea	Crab, crayfish, langostinos, lobster, prawns, shrimp
Flatfish	Butterfish, dab, dollar fish, flounder, fluke, halibut, petrale, plaice, rax, sanddab, sole, sole turbot
Fungus/Fungi	Baker's yeast, brewer's yeast, molds in cheese, mushroom, puffballs, truffle
Ginger/Zingiberaceae	Cardamon, East Indian arrowroot, ginger, turmeric
Goosefoot/ Chenopodiaceae	Beet, beet sugar, lamb's quarters, orach, spinach, Swiss chard
Gourd/Melon/ Ucurbitaceae	*Cucumbers, pickles, melons*: canary, cantaloupe, casaba, crenshaw, honeydew, Persian, watermelon; *squash*: acorn, butternut, gherkin, hubbard, pattypan, pumpkin, spaghetti, summer zucchini
Grains/Gluten/ Gramineae	Barley, kamut, malt, oat, pumpernickel, rye, spelt, triticale, wheat
Grains/Grasses	Bamboo shoots, corn, lemon grass, millet, milo, molasses, rice, sorghum, sugar cane, wild rice
Grape/Vitaceae	Currants (commercial), grape, raisin
Heath/Ericaceae	Bearberry, bilberry, blueberry, cranberry, huckleberry
Laurel/Lauraceae	Avocado, bay leaf, camphor, cinnamon, gumbo file, sassafras

Legume/Pea/	
Leguminosae	*Alfalfa, beans*: adzuki, black turtle, carob, fava, garbanzo, great northern, green, kidney, lentil, lima, lupine, masur, mung, navy, peanut, pinto, purple-hull, snap, soy, split, string; *peas*: blackeyed, chick, cream, crowder, fenugreek field, guar gum, gum acacia, kudzu
Lily/Liliaceae	Asparagus, chives, garlic, green onions, leeks, onions, sarsaparilla, shallots
Mackerel/	
Scombroidea	Albacore, bonito, mackerel, marlin, pompano, sailfish, shipjack, swordfish, tuna, yellowtail
Madder/Rubiaceae	Coffee
Mint/Labiatae	Basil, bergamot, betony, catnip, chia, clary, horehound, hyssop, lemon balm, marjoram, menthol, mint, oregano, peppermint, rosemary, sage, savory, spearmint, summer savory, thyme
Mollusk/Mollusca	Abalone, clams, cockle, mussels, octopus, oyster, scallops, snail, squid
Morning Glory/	
Convolvulaceae	Camote, jicama, sweet potato
Mustard/Cruciferae	Broccoli, brussels sprouts, cabbage, cabbage kraut, canola, cauliflower, Chinese cabbage, collards, cress, horseradish, kale, kohlrabi, mustard, radish, rutabaga, turnip, watercress
Myrtle/Myrtaceae	Allspice, clove, guava, Jamaica pepper, mace, nutmeg
Nightshade/Potato/	
Lanaceae	Eggplant, potato, tomato, peppers: cayenne, chili, green, hot, jalapeño, paprika, pimento, red, tomatillo,
Olive/Oleaceae	*Olives*: black, green, ripe; olive oil
Orchid/Orchidaceae	Vanilla
Parsley/Umbelliferae	Anise, caraway, carrot, celeria, celery seed, chervil, cilantro, coriander, cumin, dill, fennel, lovage, parsley, parsnip

Pepper/Piperaceae	Black pepper, peppercorns, white pepper
Pheasant/Phasianidae	Chicken, Cornish hen, egg white, egg yolk, pheasant, quail, seafowl
Pineapple/ Bromeliaceae	Bromelain, pineapple
Rose/Rosaceae	Almond, apricot, apple, blackberry, boysenberry, cherry, crabapple, dewberry, loganberry, loquat, nectarine, peach, pear, plum, prune, quince, raspberry, rose hips, strawberry, wild cherry
Salmon/Salmonidae	Salmon, steelhead, smelt, trout, whitefish
Sesame/Pedaliaceae	Sesame seeds
Swine/Suidae	Bacon, ham, pig, pork, swine
Tea/Theaceae	Black tea, green tea, orange pekoe, pekoe
Turkey/Meleagrididae	Turkey, turkey eggs
Yams/Dioscoreaceae	Black yams, Chinese potato, cush-cush, elephants' foot, yampee, yams, water yams, yellow yams

Detailed Food Family Index

Biologists and zoologists who study plants and animals have an extensive food family index that further identifies food-family similarities. Because foods may cross react with another member of their food family if too much is consumed, this detailed list may be helpful to people who have severe allergic symptoms.

Food Families of the Plant Kingdom

Arrowroot	West Indian arrowroot
Banana	Common bananas, dwarf banana, gros michel, plantains
Beet	Beet sugar, common beet, spinach, sugar beet, Swiss chard
Buckwheat	Rhubarb, buckwheat
Carrot	Angelica, anise, caraway, carrot, celery, celery seed, dill, fennel, parsley, parsnip

Cashew	Cashew nut, pistachio nut, mango
Chestnut	Beechnuts: American, European, Spanish; chestnuts: American, Chinese, Spanish
Chicle	Chicle
Chocolate	Chocolate, cocoa, cola, gum karaya
Citrus	Citron, common orange, grapefruit, kumquat, lemon, lime, Mandarin orange, sour orange, tangerine
Coffee	Coffee
Composite	Chamomile, chicory, common artichoke, dandelion, endive, escarole, goldenrod, lettuce (leaf and head), oyster plant, safflower, sunflower
Elderberry	Elderberry
Fungus	Bacterial cultures (yogurt, kefir, cheeses), commercial mushroom, common wild mushroom, yeast (alcoholic beverages, vinegar, vitamins)
Ginger	Ginger, turmeric
Ginseng	American ginseng, Asian ginseng
Gooseberry	Currant, gooseberry
Grape	Baking powder, cream of tartar, muscadine grape, raisin, slip-skin grape, Wine grape
Grass	Bamboo, barley, browntop, corn (corn starch, corn oil, corn syrup, cerulose, dextrose, glucose), millet, oats, rice, sorghum, sugar cane (sucrose, sugar, molasses), wheat (flour, patent flour, gluten, graham flour, bran, wheat germ), wild oats
Heath	Blueberries, cranberries, huckleberries, wintergreen
Jerusalem Artichoke	Jerusalem Artichoke
Jicama	Jicama
Laurel	Avocado, cinnamon, sassafras
Legume	Bush bean, broad bean, carob, chick pea, cowpea, gum acacia, gum tragacanth, kidney bean, lentil,

	licorice, lima bean, navy bean, pea, peanut, peanut oil, pigeon pea, soybean (flour, oil, lecithin), Spanish pea, string bean, Windsor bean
Lily	Asparagus, chives, garlic, leek, onion, Welsh onion, yucca
Litchi Nut	Litchi nut
Lotus	Chinese lotus
Macadamia Nut	Chinese yam, Indian yam, macadamia nuts
Mallow	Okra, cottonseed oil
Maple	Maple syrup
Mulberry	Breadfruit, common fig, hops
Mustard	Bok choy, broccoli, brussel sprouts, cauliflower, Chinese cabbage, collards, common cabbage, horseradish, kale, kohlrabi, mustard, radish, rutabaga, savoy cabbage, turnip
Myrtle	Allspice, clove, guava
Nightshade	Basil, cayenne, chili peppers, Chinese artichoke, eggplant, garden peppers, horehound, lavender, marjoram, potato, rosemary, sage, savory, thyme, tobacco, tomato
Nutmeg	Mace, true nutmeg
Orchid	Vanilla
Palm	Coconut, date palm, sago
Papaya	Papaya
Pawpaw	American pawpaw
Pepper	Black pepper
Persimmon	Persimmon
Pineapple	Pineapple
Rose	Almond, apple (apple cider, vinegar, apple pectin), apricot, blackberry, peach, pear, plum, prune, raspberry, sour cherries, strawberry, sweet cherries
Sarsaparilla	Sarsaparilla
Squash	Cantaloupe, Casaba, cucumber, honeydew, Indian gherkin, large pumpkin, muskmelon,

pumpkin, Persian melon, Spanish melon,
summer squash, watermelon, winter squash

Sweet Potato	Sweet potato
Tapioca	Cassava, tapioca, yucca
Taro	Malanga, poi, taro, yuatia
Tea	Tea
Walnut	Black walnut, butternut, English walnut, hickory, hinds black walnut, pecans, white walnut
Water Chestnut	Chinese water chestnut
Yam	Tropical yam

Food Families of the Animal Kingdom

Alligator	American
Antelope	Pronghorn antelope
Bear	Brown bear, black bear, grizzly bear, polar bear
Beaver	Beaver
Bovine	American bison, American buffalo, beef, Brahman, cow milk (yogurt, cottage cheese, cheese, kefir, buttermilk, butter, whey), gelatin, goat milk (cheese, yogurt), lamb (mutton, goat), rennin, sheep, sheep cheese, veal
Buffalo	Bigmouth buffalo, black buffalo, sucker
Butterfish	Butterfish
Camel	Arabian, Bactrian, llama
Carp	Carp
Cat	Lion, tiger
Catfish	Catfish, Mississippi catfish, Yellow bullhead
Chicken	Chicken eggs, domestic chicken, domestic pheasant, Indian pheasant, peafowl, quail
Cod	Atlantic cod, haddock, pollack, silver hake, tomcod
Conger Eel	Conger eel
Croaker	Atlantic croaker, freshwater drumfish, king whiting, weakfish
Decapods	Crab, crayfish, lobster, prawn, shrimp

Deer	American elk, caribou, European red deer, moose, reindeer, white-tailed deer
Dolphin Fish	Dolphin fish
Duck	Duck, duck eggs, goose, goose eggs
Eel	Common eel: European, North American
Elephant	Asiatic, African
Frog	American bullfrog, European edible bullfrog
Giraffe	Common giraffe, Somali giraffe
Green Turtle	Green turtle
Grouse	Grouse, prairie chicken
Guinea Fowl	Guinea fowl
Guinea Pig	Domestic guinea pig
Hippopotamus	Hippopotamus
Horse	Horse
Left-Eyed Flounder	California halibut, southern flounder, summer flounder
Mollusks	cephalopods (squid), gastropods (abalone, snail), pelecypods (clam, mussel, oyster, scallop)
Mullet	Gray mullet, silversides, striped mullet, white bait, white mullet
Muskrat	Muskrat
Ocean Perch	Rosefish, ocean perch
Opossum	Opossum
Pig	Pig (pork, ham, sausage)
Pigeon	Pigeon, pigeon eggs
Porgy	Porgy
Puffer	Puffer
Rabbit	Belgian hare, domestic guinea pig, domestic rabbit, Eastern cottontail, jack rabbit, showshoe rabbit, Western cottontail
Raccoon	Raccoon
Rattler	Eastern diamondback, Western diamondback
Right-Eyed Flounder	Atlantic halibut, Pacific halibut, winter flounder
Sea Lion	Sea Lion
Sea Robin	Sea robins, sea tags
Seal	Common seal

Snapping Turtle	Snapping turtle
Sole	Common sole, European sole
Squirrel	Fox squirrel, gray squirrel, red squirrel, prairie dog, woodchuck
Terrapin	Diamondback terrapin
Tuna	Atlantic mackerel, Atlantic bonito, bluefish tuna, chili bonito, frigate mackerel, king mackerel, skipjack tuna, Spanish mackerel
Turkey	Turkey, turkey eggs
Walrus	Walrus
Whale and Dolphin	Ten families
Wolf	Wolf

Appendix C

Nutritional Comparison of Selected Flours

	Calories	Protein	B₆	Folic Acid	Pantothenic Acid
Amaranth	729	28	.44	95	2
Buckwheat	402	15	.70	64	.5
Cornmeal, enriched	506	12	.35	66	.4
Quinoa	636	22	NA	NA	NA
Rice flour, brown	574	11.4	1.6	25	2.5
Rice flour, sweet white	578	9.4	.69	6	1.3
Rice flour, dark	415	18	.57	77	1.9
Rice flour, white	374	8.6	.24	23	.68
Wheat flour, whole wheat	407	16.4	.41	52	1.2
Wheat flour, white	455	12.9	.06	33	.55

	Magnesium	Zinc	Copper	Manganese
Amaranth	518	6	1.5	4.4
Buckwheat	301	4	.61	2.4
Cornmeal, enriched	56	.9	.10	.14
Quinoa	178	2.8	.7	NA
Rice flour, brown	177	3.9	.36	6.3
Rice flour, sweet white	55	1.3	.21	1.9
Rice flour, dark	318	7.2	.96	8.6
Rice flour, white	72	1.8	.26	2.0
Wheat flour, whole wheat	166	3.5	.46	4.6
Wheat flour, white	27	.88	.18	.853

This table provides a comparison of key nutrients in one cup of various grains. Each grain has its own unique nutritional profile. The less refined the flour is (whole wheat versus white wheat), the higher the nutritional levels for vitamin B_6, folic acid, pantothenic acid, magnesium, zinc, copper, and manganese. Use whole grain flours whenever possible for maximum nutrition.

Appendix D
Flour Substitutions

Various flours can be substituted for 1 cup of wheat flour in recipes. Flour substitutions tend to work best in cookie and muffin recipes rather than bread and cake recipes. Here are some substitutions for 1 cup of wheat flour.

1 cup corn flour
¾ cup coarse cornmeal
¾ cup cornstarch
6/8 cup potato flour
⅞ cup buckwheat
⅞ cup rice flour
1⅓ cups ground rolled oats
1⅛ cups oat flour
¾ cup soybean flour
1 cup barley
1 cup millet
1¼ cups rye flour
1 cup tapioca flour
½ cup arrowroot starch
1 cup teff flour
¾ cup spelt flour

You can also combine different types of flour to equal 1 cup of wheat flour

½ cup rye flour + ⅓ cup potato flour
⅓ cup rye flour + ⅝ cup rice flour
1 cup soy flour + ¾ cup potato flour
⅝ cup rice flour + ⅓ cup potato flour

½ cup cornstarch + ½ cup rye flour
½ cup cornstarch + ½ cup potato flour

Thickeners

To replace 1 tablespoon of wheat flour in soups, sauces, gravies, and puddings, use one of the following:

½ tablespoon cornstarch
½ tablespoon potato starch
½ tablespoon rice flour
½ tablespoon arrowroot
2 teaspoons quick-cooking tapioca
2 tablespoons uncooked rice
½ tablespoon lima bean flour
½ tablespoon gelatin
1 tablespoon tapioca flour
1 egg

Appendix E

Food Sources of Vinegar

Vinegar has been used for more than 10,000 years, but in food-allergy diets the use of vinegar is controversial. There are complex reasons for this. Although the first vinegars were discovered when a cask of wine had passed its time, modern technology has sought to speed up the fermentation process and alter the source of the sugar used.

The most common sources of vinegar are apples (cider vinegar), ethyl alcohol (distilled vinegar), and malt. But other fermentable sources can be used—fruits, grains, and berries. Not all vinegars are labeled with the fermentable source used, and this may create problems for food-allergy sufferers. Look closely at the ingredient label to try and identify the food source.

Distilled vinegar or grain vinegar has a grain source. Corn is the most inexpensive source frequently used but other grains, grain mashes, and cereal sludge can be used as the major ingredient in the feeder stock for yeasts in the fermentation process.

Cider vinegar is made from the juice of apples.

Malt vinegar uses malt barley and/or other cereal grains as the fermentation material. The malting process breaks down proteins into peptides; however, some people with grain/gluten sensitivities may experience symptoms after ingesting malt vinegar.

Balsamic vinegar is made from the juice of grapes in a lengthy fermentation process. No grain or grain products are used in traditional balsamic vinegars that carry the API (Association of Italian Producers of Vinegar) designation.

"Kosher for Passover" vinegars are grain- and gluten-free by definition since no grains are allowed during this time.

Appendix F

Special Food Suppliers

Allergy Resources
P. O. Box 264
Brookridge, Palmer Lake, CO 80133
Phone (800) USE FLAX. www.allergyresources.com
Assortment of foods

Arrowhead Mills, Inc.
Box 2059
Hereford, TX 79045
Phone (800) 749-0730.
Amaranth, barley, buckwheat, kamut, millet, quinoa, rice,
spelt flours

Dietary Specialties, Inc.
P. O. Box 227
Rochester, NY
Phone (800) 544-0099. www.dietspec.com
Gluten-free foods: pasta, crackers, bread, flavoring
extracts, cookies
Baking and cooking ingredients: rice flour, potato starch,
tapioca flour, xantham gum, guar gum
Baking mixes: cakes, bread, muffins, brownies

Eden Foods, Inc.
701 Tecumseh Rd.
Clinton, MI 49236
Phone (800) 248-0320, fax (517) 456-6075.
Organic and natural food products

Ener-G Foods, Inc.
P. O. Box 84487
Seattle, WA 98124-5787
Phone (800) 331-5222. www.ener-g.com
Gluten-free foods and baking mixes, poi (Hawaiian
    taro root)

Purity Foods, Inc.
2871 W. Jolly Rd.
Okemos, MI 48864
Phone (800) 997-7358, fax (517) 351-9391.
    www.purityfoods.com
Spelt flour and products, rice, wild rice, soy flour

Special Foods
9207 Shotgun Ct.
Springfield, VA 22152
Phone (703) 644-0991. www.specialfoods.com
Cassava, malanga, yam, lotus, amaranth, quinoa, and
    many other flours, baking powders

REFERENCES

Achkar, E., R. G. Farmer, B. Fleshler. "Food Allergy." *Clinical Gastroenterology*, second edition. Philadelphia: Lea & Febiger, 1992.

Agata, H., N. Kondo, O. Fukutomi, S. Shinoda, and T. Orii. "Effect of Elimination Diets on Food Specific IgE Antibodies and Lymphocyte Proliferative Responses to Food Antigens in Atopic Dermatitis Patients Exhibiting Sensitivity to Food Allergens." *Journal of Allergy & Clinical Immunology*, Vol. 91, No. 2, Feb. 1993.

Boccafogli, A., L. Vincentini, A. Camerani, P. Cogliati, A. D'Ambrosi, R. Scolozzi. "Adverse Food Reactions in Patients with Grass Pollen Allergic Respiratory Disease." *Annuals of Allergy*, Vol. 73, Oct. 1994.

Breneman, J. *Basics of Food Allergies*. Springfield, IL: Charles C. Thomas, 1978.

Bushway, R. J. and T. S. Fan. "Detection of Pesticide and Drug Residues in Food by Immunoassay." *Food Technology*, Vol. 49, No. 3, Feb. 1995.

Butkus, S. N., and L. K. Mahan. "Food Allergies: Immunological Reactions to Food." *Journal of the American Dietetic Association*, Vol. 86. May 1986.

Deamer, W. C., J. W. Gerrard, and F. Speer. "Cow's Milk Allergy, a Critical Review." *Journal of Family Practice*, Vol. 2, 1979.

Denman, A. M., B. Mitchell, B. M. Ansell. "Joint Complaints and Food Allergic Disorders." *Annuals of Allergy*. 1983.

Fallstrom, S. P., S. Shlstedt, B. Carlsson, et al. "Serum Antibodies Against Native, Processed and Digested Cow's Milk Proteins in Children with Cow's Milk Protein Intolerance." *Clinical Allergy*. 1986.

Gerard, J. C. *Food Allergies, New Perspectives*. Springfield, IL: Charles C. Thomas, 1980.

Hefle, S. L. "Immunoassay Fundamentals." *Food Technology*, Vol. 49, No. 2, Feb. 1995.

Iwasaki, T., and G. Kawaniski. *Milk Intolerances and Rejections*. Basel: Karger Publishing, 1983.

James, J. M. and H. A. Sampson. "Immunologic Changes Associated with the Development of Tolerance in Children with Cow Milk Allergy." *The Journal of Pediatrics*, Vol. 21, Aug. 1992.

Johnson, A. O., J. G. Semenya, M. S. Buchowski, C. O. Enwonwu, and N. S. Scrimshaw. "Correlation of Lactose Maldigestion, Lactose Intolerance and Milk Intolerance." *The American Journal of Clinical Nutrition*, Vol. 57, March 1993.

Joint Report of the Royal College of Physicians and the British Nutrition Foundation. "Food Intolerance and Food Aversion." *Journal Royal College of Physicians*. April 1984.

Joneja, J. V. *Managing Food Allergy and Intolerance: A Practical Guide*. West Vancouver, Canada: McQuaid Consulting Group, 1995.

Kemeny, R. D., R. Urbanek, P. L. Amlot, et al. "Subclass of IgG in Allergic Disease, IgG Subclass Antibodies in Immediate and Non-immediate Food Allergy." *Clinical Allergy*. 1986.

Lessof, M. H., D. M. Kemeny. "Non IgE Mediated Reactions to Food: How Much is Allergic." *Annual of Allergy*. 1987.

Metcalfe, D. D., H. A. Sampson, R. A. Simon. *Food Allergy: Adverse Reactions to Foods and Food Additives*. Cambridge, MA: Second Ed. Blackwell Science, 1997.

Miller, J. B. *Food Allergy: Provocative Testing and Injection Therapy*. Springfield, IL: Charles C. Thomas, 1972.

"MSG: A Pervasive and Hidden Danger in Your Food Supply." *Dr. Sherry Rogers' Total Health in Today's World*. Vol. 1, No. 6, Sept. 1997.

Nordlee, J. A. and S. L. Taylor. "Immunological Analysis of Food Allergens and Other Food Proteins." *Food Technology*, Vol. 49, No. 3, Feb. 1995.

Perkin, J. E. *Food Allergies and Adverse Reaction*. Gaithersburg, MD: Aspen Publishers, 1990.

Philpott, W. and W. K. Kalita. *Brain Allergies*. New Canaan, CT: Keats Publishing Co., 1980.

Rafei, A., S. Peters, N. Harris, and J. Bellani. "Food Allergy and Food Specific IgG Measurements." *Annuals of Allergy*. 1989.

Randolph, T. G., and R. W. Moss. *Allergies—Your Hidden Enemy*. NY: Lippincott & Crowell, 1980.

Ranhotra, G. S., J. A. Gelroth, B. K. Glaser, and K. J. Lorenz. "Nutrient Composition of Spelt Wheat." *Journal of Food Composition and Analysis*, Vol. 9, March 1996.

Ranhotra, G. S., J. A. Gelroth, B. K. Glaser, K. J. Lorenz, and D. L. Johnson. "Composition and Protein Nutritional Quality of Quinoa." *Cereal Chemistry*, Vol. 70, May/June 1993.

Rapp, D. *Allergies and Your Family*. NY: Sterling Publishing, 1980.

Rowe, A. H. *Food Allergy, Its Manifestations, Diagnosis and Treatment*. Philadelphia: Lea and Febiger, 1931.

Sampson, H. A., and D. D. Metcalfe. "Primer on Allergic and Immunologic Diseases." *The Journal of the American Medical Association*, Vol. 268, Nov. 25, 1992.

Sandberg, D. H. "Gastrointestinal Complaints Related to Diet." *International Pediatrics*, Vol. 5, 1990.

Schmidt, M., M. H. Flock. "Food Hypersensitivity and the Irritable Bowel Syndrome." *American Journal of Gastroenterology*. 1991.

Shakib, F., H. M. Brown, A. Phelps, and R. Redhead. "Study of IgG Subclass Antibodies in Patients with Milk Intolerance." *Clinical Allergy*, Vol. 16, 1986.

Simoons, F. J. "The Geographic Hypothesis and Lactose Malabsorption: A Weighing of the Evidence." *Digestive Disease*, Vol. 23, 1978.

Taylor, S. L. "Food Allergies and Sensitivities." *Journal of the American Dietetic Association*, Vol. 86, No. 5, May 1986.

Tu, L. C., J. H. Strimas, and S. L. Bahna. "Estimated Magnitude of Food Allergy by U.S. Physicians." *Annuals of Allergy*. 1988.

Recipe Index

INDEX